Building a Culture of Patient Safety Through Simulation

Kathleen Gallo, PhD, MBA, RN, FAAN, is senior vice president and chief learning officer for the North Shore-Long Island Jewish Health System (NS-LIJ). Under her leadership, the Center for Learning and Innovation—NS-LIJ's corporate university—and the Patient Safety Institute were created to transform the health system into a learning organization by strategically focusing on workforce development. Dr. Gallo is responsible for leadership development throughout the organization. She initiated the creation and implementation of a comprehensive learning strategy, and the development of a new human resources (HR) architecture that transformed HR into a strategic business partner. Within NS-LIJ, Dr. Gallo has served as system director for emergency medicine and vice president for emergency medical services. She has more than 25 years' experience in emergency nursing, having held a variety of clinical and administrative positions in tertiary care hospitals on Long Island.

Dr. Gallo serves on the advisory boards for the Executive Program in Work-Based Learning Leadership at the University of Pennsylvania, and the Institute of Healthcare Improvement Open School for Health Professions. She is the former chair of the Quality Committee for the Council for Accreditation, Society for Simulation in Healthcare, and serves on the editorial board of the *Journal for Applied Nursing Research*. Dr. Gallo is an associate professor of science education at the Hofstra NS-LIJ School of Medicine; an associate adjunct professor at the Frances Payne Bolton School of Nursing, Case Western Reserve University; and an adjunct professor at the Bouvé College of Health Sciences, Northeastern University. She served as an examiner for the Malcolm Baldrige Quality Award Program from 2003 to 2005 and also served on the advisory board for the National Center for Healthcare Leadership (NCHL) from 2004 to 2010. In addition, she has held several regional posts for emergency medical services and emergency nursing.

A noted speaker, Dr. Gallo addresses a wide range of subjects including Future Workforce Requirements, Creating a World Class Learning Organization, Effective Leadership for Today's Workforce, Preparing Tomorrow's Clinicians for Tomorrow's Healthcare System, Enhancing Patient Safety Through Interprofessional Education and Collaboration, Heralding in a New Era: Patient Safety at the Forefront, Transforming Healthcare Into Higher Reliability Organizations, and Creating a Culture of Safety: Lessons Learned from Aviation.

Dr. Gallo is a board member of the American Nurses Foundation Board of Trustees, the National Advisory Council on Nurse Education and Practice for the U.S. Department of Health and Human Services, National Advisory Council for the National Center of Interprofessional Practice and Education, the American Association of Colleges of Nursing Futures Task Force, the Advisory Council for Career and Technical Education for the New York City Department of Education, and the Commission on Accreditation of Healthcare Management Education. Dr. Gallo was inducted as a fellow in the American Academy of Nursing in 2011. She was also inducted into the 2005 Hall of Fame at Adelphi University School of Nursing, and received the 2005 Distinguished Alumni Award from State University of New York at Stony Brook.

Dr. Gallo received her bachelor of science in nursing from Excelsior College, University of the State of New York; a master of science (nursing) degree from the State University of New York at Stony Brook; a PhD (nursing) from Adelphi University, Garden City, New York; and a master in business administration, also from Adelphi University.

Lawrence G. Smith, MD, MACP, is the physician-in-chief of the North Shore-Long Island Jewish Health System (NS-LIJ) and founding dean of the Hofstra North Shore-LIJ School of Medicine. Dr. Smith joined NS-LIJ in May 2005, as chief academic officer and senior vice president of academic affairs and then served as the Health System's chief medical officer, prior to his current role. Dr. Smith earned his medical degree from New York University School of Medicine, along with a bachelor of science degree in physics from Fordham University. His residency in internal medicine at Strong Memorial Hospital was followed by military service as captain in the Army Medical Corps at Fitzsimmons Army Medical Center in Denver, Colorado. He practiced general internal medicine at SUNY Stony Brook, where he served as director of education and program director of the residency in internal medicine for 6 years. For the next 11 years, at Mount Sinai School of Medicine in Manhattan, he served as dean and chairman of medical education, founder and director of the school's Institute for Medical Education, professor of medicine, and an attending physician. Prior to his appointment as dean at Mount Sinai, Dr. Smith had been vice chair of medicine and program director of the Internal Medicine Residency.

He is a national leader in medical education with many peer-reviewed publications and national presentations. He is a former member of the board of directors of the American Board of Internal Medicine and has served in multiple capacities in the Association of Program Directors of Internal Medicine, including president. He is a former governor and a former regent of the American College of Physicians. In April 2011, he was awarded Mastership of the American College of Physicians. Dr. Smith is a member-at-large of the National Board of Medical Examiners and a member of the New York Academy of Medicine. He serves on the Executive Committee of the Associated Medical Schools of New York (AMSNY) and on the Advisory Committee on Long-Term Clinical Clerkships for the New York State Education Department.

Building a Culture of Patient Safety Through Simulation

An Interprofessional Learning Model

Kathleen Gallo, PhD, MBA, RN, FAAN
Lawrence G. Smith, MD, MACP
Editors

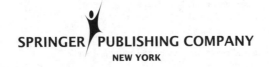

SPRINGER PUBLISHING COMPANY
NEW YORK

Springer Publishing Company, LLC
11 West 42nd Street
New York, NY 10036
www.springerpub.com

Acquisitions Editor: Joseph Morita
Production Editor: Brian Black
Composition: S4Carlisle Publishing Services

ISBN: 978-0-8261-6906-8
e-book ISBN: 978-0-8261-6907-5

14 15 16 17 / 5 4 3 2 1

The author and the publisher of this Work have made every effort to use sources believed to be reliable to provide information that is accurate and compatible with the standards generally accepted at the time of publication. Because medical science is continually advancing, our knowledge base continues to expand. Therefore, as new information becomes available, changes in procedures become necessary. We recommend that the reader always consult current research and specific institutional policies before performing any clinical procedure. The author and publisher shall not be liable for any special, consequential, or exemplary damages resulting, in whole or in part, from the readers' use of, or reliance on, the information contained in this book. The publisher has no responsibility for the persistence or accuracy of URLs for external or third-party Internet websites referred to in this publication and does not guarantee that any content on such websites is, or will remain, accurate or appropriate.

Library of Congress Cataloging-in-Publication Data

Building a culture of patient safety through simulation : an interprofessional learning model / Kathleen Gallo, Lawrence G. Smith, editors.
     p. ; cm.
  Includes bibliographical references and index.
  ISBN 978-0-8261-6906-8 (alk. paper)—ISBN 0-8261-6906-6 (alk. paper)—ISBN 978-0-8261-6907-5 (e-book)
  I. Gallo, Kathleen, editor. II. Smith, Lawrence G., editor.
  [DNLM: 1. Patient Safety. 2. Interprofessional Relations. 3. Organizational Culture. 4. Patient Care Team. 5. Teaching—methods. WX 185]
  R729.8
  610.28'9—dc23
                         2014016815

Special discounts on bulk quantities of our books are available to corporations, professional associations, pharmaceutical companies, health care organizations, and other qualifying groups. If you are interested in a custom book, including chapters from more than one of our titles, we can provide that service as well.

For details, please contact:
Special Sales Department, Springer Publishing Company, LLC
11 West 42nd Street, 15th Floor, New York, NY 10036-8002
Phone: 877-687-7476 or 212-431-4370; Fax: 212-941-7842
E-mail: sales@springerpub.com

Printed in the United States of America by McNaughton & Gunn.

As an expert in aviation simulation, having created globally recognized programs for the U.S. Navy and JetBlue Airways, I am inspired by the visionary leaders at North Shore-LIJ who have made such a remarkable commitment to improving performance outcomes across their system through simulation.

Mike Barger, EdD
Co-Founder, Chief Learning Officer, Captain, JetBlue Airways
Former Chief Training Officer, United States Navy Fighter Weapons School (TOPGUN)

Simulated learning provides a safe environment for testing new behaviors and skills. This book is a timely and much needed resource that will serve as a guide to educating new and existing members of all health professions. I think it should be required reading for anyone seeking to drive change in health care.

Geraldine Polly Bednash, PhD, RN, FAAN
Chief Executive Officer/Executive Director
American Association of Colleges of Nursing

This book will save lives. The authors generously share their journey to building a world class integration of safety tools, from simulation and communication, to team training and safety science. They show how simulation will teach new ways to see and offer insights into performance that will improve care in every part of a hospital system. Every physician, nurse, pharmacist, and student will learn and care for patients in a new way.

Maureen Bisognano
President and CEO
Institute for Healthcare Improvement

This book isn't just an inspirational story about a patient safety journey of a large health care organization. It's full of great lessons with enough detail to guide others to do the same. And, it's a virtual roadmap for how the wise and varied use of simulation can help to move the giant boulder of safety culture up the steep hill of resistance to change.

Jeffrey B. Cooper, PhD
Professor of Anaesthesia, Harvard Medical School
Department of Anaesthesia, Critical Care & Pain Medicine
Massachusetts General Hospital, Boston, Massachusetts
Executive Director, Center for Medical Simulation

This book is not fundamentally about medical simulation. Rather, it is truly about the concepts of safety and quality, coupled with health care reformation, utilizing simulation as the mechanism of organizational improvement in service to patients. The new era of safety and quality, begun by forces such as the Institute of Medicine reports, finds in this text the natural evolution of positive process change.

William F. Dunn, MD, FCCP, FCCM
Associate Professor of Medicine
Division of Pulmonary & Critical Care Medicine
Mayo Clinic
Past President, Society for Simulation in Healthcare
Past Medical Director, Mayo Clinic Multidisciplinary Simulation Center

Gallo and Smith have provided us with a definitive roadmap of how simulation can be used successfully to advance interprofessional health education for all disciplines. Focused on patient safety, the patient is, in fact, at the center of their thinking as it should be for all of us . . . . [This book] adds the theoretical underpinnings of that work that has been missing in other textbooks. I recommend it to every health educator who is interested in preparing students for the complexity of the clinical environment in order to improve safety and quality in all care.

Terry Fulmer, PhD, RN, FAAN
Dean, Bouvé College of Health Sciences, Northeastern University
Trustee, Josiah Macy Jr. Foundation

[This] is not a typical text—rather, a guide with intentional simulation learning encounters to foster and implement a culture of patient safety. Impressive in its approach, each chapter within the book uses simulation to address patient safety across the continuum of health from system-wide initiatives to combat sepsis; or respond to medical emergencies in psychiatric care, perinatal care, and pediatric care; to improve retention of members of the health care team; and improve our ability to assess and evaluate learning.

Beverly Malone, PhD, RN, FAAN
CEO, National League for Nursing

This is an important and timely book from a highly functioning, integrated health care system that also has made an enormous commitment to health professions education. The book is both practical and aspirational in detailing how interprofessional simulation can be a powerful tool to help achieve the common goals of educational reform and delivery reform—more reliable, safer, and efficient patient care.

George E. Thibault, MD
President, Josiah Macy Jr. Foundation

Contents

Contributors

Patti Adelman, LMSW
Director of the Physician Leadership Institute, Center for Learning and Innovation, Lake Success, NY

Stephen Bello, RPA-C
Vice President of Cardiovascular and Thoracic Surgery, North Shore University Hospital, Manhasset, NY

Michael Cassara, DO, FACEP, CHSE
Associate Professor of Emergency Medicine, Hofstra North Shore-LIJ School of Medicine, Medical Director, Patient Safety Institute, Associate Residency Program Director and Director of Simulation, North Shore University Hospital, Manhasset, NY

Barbara DeVoe, DNP, FNP-BC
Vice President of Interprofessional Education and Learning, North Shore-LIJ Health System, Director of the Patient Safety Institute, North Shore-LIJ Health System, Assistant Professor of Science Education, Hofstra North Shore-LIJ School of Medicine, Hempstead, NY

Martin Doerfler, MD
Associate Professor of Medicine and Science Education, Hofstra North Shore-LIJ School of Medicine, Senior Vice President, Clinical Strategy and Development, North Shore-LIJ Health System, Assistant Chief Medical Officer, North Shore-LIJ Health System, Great Neck, NY

Andrew Drozd, EMT-B
Medical Simulation Technician, Patient Safety Institute, Lake Success, NY

Adiel Fleischer, MD
Chairman of Obstetrics/Gynecology, Executive Director, Women's Health Service Line, North Shore-LIJ Health System, Great Neck, NY

M. Isabel Friedman, DNP, MPA, RN, BC, CCRN, CNN, CHSE
Director, Patient Safety Institute, Assistant Professor of Science Education, Hofstra North Shore-LIJ School of Medicine, Hempstead, NY

Kathleen Gallo, PhD, MBA, RN, FAAN
Senior Vice President and Chief Learning Officer, North Shore-LIJ Health System,
Associate Professor of Science Education, Hofstra North Shore-LIJ School
of Medicine, Hempstead, NY

Sandeep Gangadharan, MD
Assistant Professor of Pediatrics, Division of Pediatric Critical Care Medicine,
Director of Medical Simulation, Cohen Children's Medical Center of New York,
New Hyde Park, NY

Alan R. Hartman, MD, FACS, FACC, FCCP
Chairman and Senior Vice President, Cardiovascular and Thoracic Surgery,
North Shore University Hospital, Manhasset, NY

Stanley Katz, MD, FACC
Chairman and Senior Vice President, Department of Cardiology, North Shore
University Hospital, Manhasset, NY

Leah Kaufman, MD, FACOG
Residency Program Director and Associate Professor, Department of Obstetrics and
Gynecology, State University of New York Upstate Medical University, Syracuse, NY

Robert L. Kerner Jr., JD, EdD(c), RN, CEN
Assistant Director, Patient Safety Institute, Assistant Professor of Science Education,
Hofstra North Shore-LIJ School of Medicine, Hempstead, NY

Kristy Loewenstein, MSN, RN-BC, PMHNP-BC
Director of Nursing Education and Professional Development, Zucker Hillside
Hospital, Glen Oaks, NY

Helen Maliagros Scott, MD, FAAP
Assistant Professor of Pediatrics, Hofstra North Shore-LIJ School of Medicine,
Pediatric Hospitalist, Director of Hospitalist Simulation, Cohen Children's Medical
Center of New York, New Hyde Park, NY

Donna Marchant, MD, FACC, FACP
Assistant Professor of Medicine, Hofstra North Shore-LIJ School of Medicine,
Director of Cardiology Fellowship Program, North Shore University Hospital,
Manhasset, NY

Marybeth McManus MPA, BSN, RN-BC
Chief Nursing Officer, North Shore-LIJ Health System, Great Neck, NY

John Perrone BS, EMT-B
Medical Simulation Technician, Patient Safety Institute, Lake Success, NY

Barbara Rhodes, MSN, RN, CNOR
Perioperative Staff RN of the Lithotripter Unit, North Shore University Hospital,
Manhasset, NY

Kristen Rojas, MS, RN, CCRN
Senior Administrative Director, Patient Care Services, Cardiothoracic Surgery
and Critical Care, Southside Hospital, Bay Shore, NY

James Roth, BA, EMT-B
Assistant Medical Simulation Technician, Patient Safety Institute, Lake Success, NY

Andrew Rotjan, RN, CPEN, EMT-P
Clinical Education Specialist, Patient Safety Institute, Lake Success, NY

John Galbraith Simmons, MSEd
Medical Writer, Author and Independent Scholar, New York, NY

Lawrence G. Smith, MD, MACP
Executive Vice President & Physician-In-Chief, North Shore-LIJ Health System,
Dean, Hofstra North Shore-LIJ School of Medicine, Hempstead, NY

Michal Tamuz, PhD
Director, Research Health Outcomes, Patient Safety Institute, Lake Success, NY

Ronald Ulrich, BA, EMT
Senior Medical Simulation Technician, Patient Safety Institute, Lake Success, NY

Jane M. Wickey
Director of Standardized Patient Education, Clinical Skills Center, Lake Success, NY

Foreword

As I write this Foreword, I'm sitting in seat 3A on board an American Airlines flight. I have confidence in the cockpit crew because they have been through a rigorous training program, including hundreds of hours in a flight simulator. They have been steeped in a culture of crew resource management (CRM). I observed earlier how they introduced themselves to the flight attendants and to one another. They seemed relaxed and all of this was rather routine. When I return to my own academic medical center, my professional home for the past 24 years, I don't have a similar level of confidence in *our* systems. How could that possibly be?

Drs. Gallo and Smith have brought together a core group of national leaders to produce what I think is a paradigm-busting book that will help to transform education at the graduate level in medicine, nursing, and all related fields. The book speaks expertly about the high fidelity of simulation training, the need for synthetic models, and the adult learning theory behind the debrief—all of this is amazing, but I think here of patients.

In my nearly 30 years in academic medicine, regrettably, there is no single place for us to come together in a safe environment, without recrimination, to review our work as a team. If the general public had a deeper knowledge of our daily work process, they would be in shock. I first visited the North Shore-Long Island Jewish (LIJ) Patient Safety Institute (PSI) back in 2009, 4 years after it opened. The history of PSI is covered in detail in the pages that follow. We learn that it was an outgrowth of the Center for Learning and Innovation, which was first created in 2002, following the early formation of the North Shore-LIJ Health System around 2000. Having grown up 20 minutes south of both the North Shore and LIJ Hospitals, I never thought that in my adult life they would come together to create the current powerhouse that they represent. Nor did I ever think possible that they would build their own medical school known to the world now as the Hofstra North Shore-LIJ School of Medicine, which opened its doors officially in 2011.

So for me, this book is not only a "paradigm buster" for education in the health professions, but it is a manifesto about where we must go as an interprofessional team, caring for the patient of the future. Sure, they had all of the key ingredients to implement social change, starting with their charismatic leader, Michael Dowling, who recognized special characteristics in medical educators like Larry Smith and innovative nurse educators like Kathy Gallo.

All of those leaders are part of the "right recipe," but other ingredients include a willingness to collaborate with corporations, such as General Electric, and an open-mindedness to work with other leaders such as those at the Institute for Healthcare Improvement in Cambridge, Massachusetts. It is as though all the right ingredients came together with a winning recipe to build one of the most impressive simulation centers in our country.

And yet, the simulation center itself, while very impressive, is only bricks and mortar. It takes a senior-level commitment across a gigantic system like North Shore-LIJ to turn this simulation center into the "paradigm buster" that it has become. We all talk about learning organizations and the need to train our people to create a safe culture. The simulation center and the deep science that now lie behind it enable North Shore-LIJ to achieve this national leadership position, which, in turn, gave rise to this winning book.

Again, to me it is all very personal. Not only were these hospitals looming large in my adolescence, but as a national leader myself, in the movement to bring quality and safety into the mainstream of medical education, my in-person visits to PSI played a seminal role in my thinking. That is, while the technology is impressive, the culture is even more so. Imagine the following scenario: There is a difficult delivery of a preterm infant at a North Shore-LIJ member hospital and the team members are very upset about a poor outcome. Weeks later, this same team, in a completely safe environment, free from any recrimination, can come together under the expert leadership of Dr. Gallo and her team to evaluate what went wrong. Essentially, they do an "autopsy" on the cultural failure that led to the poor clinical outcome. How many organizations can make a similar claim? Not only does the simulation center practice this kind of task-based learning, but Drs. Gallo and Smith have taken this to the next level, whereby they practice cultural change, implement cultural change, and teach cultural change to the nation at large.

How will we know if this book is successful? I think there are several metrics. Certainly, I'm paying close attention to the Hofstra North Shore-LIJ School of Medicine. I'm hoping that its graduates will be the future proselytizers; they will be the "teach the teacher" model for the use of simulation training to improve quality and safety. That will be a key educational metric.

Another metric of success might be the quick adoption of this book as a how-to manual to move most of the nation's simulation centers from task-based learning to cultural change and the tools for creating such change. The final metric might be that this book becomes obsolete in 3 to 5 years. Meaning, we'll look back on 2014 as the inflection point in our understanding of the power of CRM. In 5 years we'll say, "Wow, that was the time when the science of simulation training was powerful enough to alter hundreds of years of clinical culture—the culture of 'see one, do one, teach one' without any real evaluation of the 'one.'"

I'm grateful to Drs. Gallo and Smith and their colleagues for putting together such a volume. The chapters have a comfortable flow and even a novice reader new to CRM will grasp the key concepts quite readily. Perhaps Drs. Gallo and Smith have actually stumbled on a new type of Flexner report; one that will have a dramatic impact on medical and nursing education for the 21st century. Here I speak of patients. Future patients will be similarly grateful for the work of these authors and contributors.

I am truly privileged to have visited this award-winning institution and to count their leaders among my professional colleagues and friends.

David B. Nash, MD, MBA
Dean, Jefferson School of Population Health
Philadelphia, Pennsylvania

Foreword

Viewed as an organizational imperative, patient safety is an aspect of quality of care. Today, aided by increasingly powerful abilities to track and evaluate the care we provide, and implement incentives to ensure optimal treatment, the business case for safety is that if you take the right steps in the right order the first time, the outcome will be better and ultimately cost effective. Although health care is more complex than other industries, and people are not machines, the best result will be the most efficient—and therein we find the case for extensive, system-wide use of simulation. If the series of initiatives detailed in this book share a common basis, it may be found in the long-term effort to instill and nurture in our organization a culture of continuous learning.

A forthright examination of any health care system in the United States at the beginning of the 21st century would show that without question its most valuable asset is the people it employs—at all levels and on all fronts—to make it work. Employees present the greatest potential, from a business standpoint, for producing value and enabling successful evolution in a rapidly changing marketplace. If organized with some understanding of the steps people at all levels can take to enhance their capabilities, education from within can generate a return on investment rather than a drain on resources. Infrastructure is always aging and requires maintenance and renewal; technology is constantly advancing in complexity and requires constant upgrades. But the capability to improve an organization committed to caring for and treating other human beings, and keeping them well, resides in the employees who, in whatever capacity, provide that care. These include not only physicians and nurses but all individuals whose work and intelligence can detect opportunities for improvement, target efficiencies, and ensure that every patient's experience embodies the highest possible quality of care.

The crucial importance of the workforce and the individual and collective roles of people in creating leadership to drive cultural change represented the root and branch of a series of questions that, in 2001, I posed to executive colleagues within the newly formed North Shore-Long Island Jewish Health System (NS-LIJ). In effect, the inquiry was simple: Who were the right people for the organization? How would we find them and keep them? Who would be responsible for hiring them and who was to be accountable?

My purpose in posing those questions was the vital need to respond to the powerful forces of transformation in the health care industry as a whole. Then, as today, they were inescapable: underlying social and demographic shifts; newly minted consumer demand for high-quality, affordable health care; pressures exerted by revolutionary biomedical technologies; and advances in therapeutics. On the financial side, those forces had generated impetus for the mergers through which NS-LIJ had been created and by which it was beset with grave, potentially perilous issues that would absolutely have to be resolved if it were to prosper and advance as a leader in a huge competitive marketplace. Two large tertiary-care hospitals that for decades had competed with each other were now a single entity; further acquisitions of many other hospitals completed the picture. Employee retention rates were low and, overall, patient satisfaction was not high. Located in a major metropolitan area, NS-LIJ was then a system with more than 35,000 employees that served a highly diverse patient population but lacked a shared identity. In the universe of contemporary health care economics, to simply settle for financial oversight of disparate institutions was not an attractive option, but rather, a potential recipe for failure.

Although I did not have all the answers, I sketched a plan to respond to these issues with an overarching aim: to infuse the entire organization with opportunities for meaningful learning. To foster improvement and innovation meant engaging employees on all levels and evoking and promoting leadership congruent with clear institutional values. My inclusive search for potential leaders (as distinct from managers) may have seemed idiosyncratic to some, but it was a response to the need to respond swiftly to the marketplace as a means of seeking a competitive advantage. An organization with a flexible hierarchy, with leaders seeded throughout who are purposely equipped with skills to identify problems, to devise solutions, and to adapt to new data, seemed to me essential if the organization was to succeed.

From these considerations and the concept, at first, of a "leadership institute," there emerged NS-LIJ's Center for Learning and Innovation (CLI), established in 2002. It was the first "corporate university" to be established by a health care system—many more have emerged over the past decade—and it followed the model set by General Electric (GE) and emulated by other corporations, such as Motorola and IBM. I had spent time at GE's Crotonville Institute and was able to recruit both that company and the Harvard School of Public Health as strategic partners—with others, both corporations and universities, to follow. Each helped to formulate educational methodologies, devise courses for a broad range of management topics and clinical domains, and to implement curricula.

Most importantly, CLI was not meant to be a "training" branch of the health care system, separate from its everyday operations. It was designed to be central to NS-LIJ and its employees: to provide opportunities for focused, meaningful learning and, at the same time, to serve as a central platform to inaugurate culture change and ultimately bring about an integrated health care system. In addition to course offerings and programs for adult learning and enrichment, we developed leadership pedagogies for physicians and nurses, and introduced process improvement methodologies such as Six Sigma and Lean, with the intention of engaging the employees' creativity throughout the system. CLI grew exponentially: from a single classroom in 2002 to 3,000 employee-students in 2004, and 15,000 by 2007. In 2013, to apply the current standard, the NS-LIJ workforce engaged in more than 265,000 learning hours in the course of the year.

One decision I made helped pave the way for the Patient Safety Institute, founded under the aegis of CLI. Just because part of my larger purpose intended to avoid the narrow scope of training courses that most health care organizations provide their employees—often, it seems, as nothing more than a way of filling their days—I appointed a chief learning officer (CLO) whom I also tasked with overseeing what I viewed as the fairly anachronistic domain of Human Resources. Purposely seeking someone not imbued with received wisdom from the world of education, but an executive who could also participate in developing a complex matrix management system, I chose, from within NS-LIJ, Kathleen Gallo.

Originally an emergency and trauma nurse with a degree in business administration and a PhD in nursing, Kathy brought me the suggestion that CLI investigate the use of simulation with a view to improving patient safety. That idea, if it could be put into practice, represented a clinical focus that would wholly align with our business aim of generating efficiencies throughout the system. At the time—this was 2005—simulation was beginning to make substantial inroads in health care. Its hands-on quality made it ideal to serve purposes of both learning and assessment while, at the same time, by addressing safety issues, it could improve the experience of providers and patients alike.

In creating the Patient Safety Institute, we had the express aim of making simulation not a one-off research project or an ancillary department—hence its name. It was not to be a standalone flavor of the month but constitute part of the institutional DNA that equates with quality. Viewed as a means to an end, we thought that simulation could become integral to an organization in the sense that quality of care is everybody's job and affects everything they do. The framework of supporting ideas bears this out: interprofessional teamwork that flattens the traditional top-down hierarchy, purposeful learning that does not treat adults like children, and emotional and intellectual engagement through hands-on experience and debriefing. Simulation represents an investment in human capital that may be expected to provide the whole organization, and the consumers of health care who frequent it, with substantial and long-term dividends.

Finally, allow me to say something about what to me seems the most attractive aspect of simulation for patient safety—and that, in a word, is its appeal to flexibility and adaptability to today's complex clinical realities. The forms it takes—with high-fidelity simulators, standardized patients, or both—provides learners with new dimensions and prospects that are not found in slide presentations, outdated didactics, or multiple-choice exams. Rather, the rational limits of simulation are formed by the application of scientific knowledge and the art and science of caring for patients; within those boundaries may be found great room for imagination and the play of ideas.

In the era we are about to enter, in which brick-and-mortar hospitals will not be where most patients will receive care, interprofessional education through simulation will reward organizations that employ it with insight and creativity. In years to come, we anticipate more and more care will be dispensed in outpatient and ambulatory facilities, in patients' homes or in settings such as hospice. Simulation has unlimited potential for introducing caregivers to these venues, for helping to detect threats to safety, and for adapting new treatment modalities of all kinds. In brief, people and organizations that can adapt and use simulation for patient safety will be prepared to lead and succeed in the complex and always surprising future of health care.

Michael J. Dowling
President and Chief Executive Officer
North Shore-LIJ Health System

Preface

Today, the drive to improve patient safety is a worldwide movement, an educational and clinical priority of global significance (Donaldson & Philip, 2004). In the 15 years since publication of *To Err Is Human* raised alarm over the extent of preventable harm, efforts to improve safety have spawned both a vast literature and a host of programmatic efforts (Kohn, Corrigan, & Donaldson, 2000). Widespread awareness has replaced tacit understanding that health care is a high-risk industry. As a field, patient safety is characterized by numerous projects and protocols, concepts and ideas, principles, approaches, and initiatives. Unfortunately, there is considerable distance between rhetoric and exhortation on one hand, and substantive advances on the other. Simulation and interprofessional learning work hand-in-hand to close that gap. Together they can help build a culture of safety that reaches across all clinical domains and all venues for learning.

Our goal at the Patient Safety Institute (PSI) of the North Shore-LIJ Health System (NS-LIJ), the genesis of which is described in Chapter 1, is to provide clients and stakeholders with a consistent process and set of options for pursuing simulation that will correspond with their larger aim of improving safety. The PSI, inaugurated in 2006, forms part of an expanding health system's concerted effort to reimagine and reshape itself as a learning organization—defined as an entity in which "people continually expand their capacity to create the results they truly desire, where new and expansive patterns of thinking are nurtured, where collective aspiration is set free, and where people are continually learning to see the whole together" (Senge, 1990, p. 3).

Our contention, expressed throughout this book, is that when simulation is strategically employed—that is, aligned with the unique requirements and larger goals of the health care system—it functions to concretely implement a culture of patient safety. It lends substance and body to the organization's "collective aspiration." Simulation employed in this way is a disruptive innovation that introduces major changes in the way that health providers communicate, with both patients and one another, for both learning and assessment; it creates advantages in the way people acquire competencies, put scientific knowledge to use, and affect treatment outcomes. It places great emphasis on principles of adult learning and work in interprofessional teams, all with a view to ensuring safety, detecting threats, and ultimately providing efficient care. Used in this way, simulation introduces a "new value proposition" (Christensen, Anthony, & Roth, 2004, p. xvii) that creates competencies and prioritizes safety.

Although PSI has evolved into a large center within a corporate university, it began in a single unused hospital room. We wish to emphasize that interprofessional learning through simulation is a scalable enterprise. Success is not about size. Health care systems of any magnitude can benefit from simulation if they deploy it in planned, strategic ways that connect aims with overall organizational goals. Effective simulation does not require the most sophisticated technology or elaborate props, but it does demand commitment to interprofessional learning and a well-trained faculty versed in the tenets of adult, experiential learning, and deliberate practice. To be effective, simulation also requires commitment to extensive debriefing that ensures learning takes place in a context that allows reflection, improved teamwork, and self-discovery. Equally important are organizational support and committed, mission-driven leadership.

USING THIS BOOK

Each chapter in this book addresses discrete aspects of simulation in the larger context of patient safety. Unlike a textbook that elucidates specialized areas for specific didactic purposes, we have devised content that will be relevant to health care professionals of all specialties. Chapters are interdisciplinary by design and composition, with a view to helping individuals and groups learn from one another.

Of the introductory chapters that comprise Part One, we provide in Chapter 1 a narrative account of the origins of PSI that emphasizes its integration and alignment with the strategic goals of the larger health care system— an example, in effect, of innovation that, from within the organization, creates new capabilities. No aspect of simulation is more central to successful application than debriefing, and Chapter 2 elaborates its historic development and evolution at PSI, offering concrete methods and examples to help show how theory translates into practical application. Chapter 3 provides an account of a system-wide initiative to combat sepsis—aligned with the international movement to stem an epidemic that costs 200,000 lives annually in North America alone; this chapter illustrates the concept of *systems integration* as representing a fourth domain of simulation, in addition to *teaching/education, assessment,* and *research* (Dunn, Deutsch, Maxworthy, Gallo, & Dong, 2013).

Accounts of interprofessional teams operating with distinct goals make up Part Two. In Chapter 4, cardiothoracic surgeon Alan Hartman and colleagues describe how they employed simulation as an organizing tool for safety and process control in advance of opening a postsurgical tertiary-grade intensive care unit in a former community hospital. In devising methods to improve the interprofessional response to acute medical emergencies in a psychiatric hospital, Kristy Loewenstein, in Chapter 5, provides an instructive example of the ways in which simulation offers distinctive advantages over simple hands-on training and code drills. Emergency physician Michael Cassara provides an in-depth summary of simulation in an emergency medicine residency program in Chapter 6.

After pioneering work in anesthesiology, pediatrics and perinatal medicine became two of the first disciplines in which providers recognized the considerable potential for simulation, as indicated by the chapters that comprise Part Three. Leah Kaufman and Adiel Fleischer explain their comprehensive effort to improve patient safety in a regional perinatal center in Chapter 7, which they tracked with a research component, and describe how they use simulation in conjunction with other long-term efforts to avoid adverse events. In Chapter 8, Sandeep Gangadharan details the way in which, for several programs in a children's hospital, each scenario serves a distinct purpose in addressing the rare acute emergencies that pediatric nurses and physicians must be prepared for, including detection of latent safety threats. Helen Scott discusses in Chapter 9 how simulation can prepare pediatric interprofessional clinical teams to contend with the common disorders seen in pediatric hospitals; she also outlines a program that employs standardized patients to improve interpersonal and communication skills among pediatrics residents.

The chapters in Part Four provide accounts of several programs that indicate both the depth and range of simulation. For a 3-year training program for cardiology residents, Donna Marchant and Stanley Katz delineate in Chapter 10 the comprehensive use of high-fidelity simulators and haptic-enhanced simulation together with standardized patients for purposes of both learning and assessment. In Chapter 11, we describe the development of a critical care nurse fellowship program that has improved retention of newly hired nurse graduates, an aim recognized as significant for patient safety; that program, initiated in 2005, proved to be in full alignment with the subsequent Institute of Medicine (IOM) recommendations by the Initiative on the Future of Nursing (2010). (The fellowship, renamed in 2007, is today the William Randolph Hearst Critical Care Nurse Fellowship Program.) In Chapter 12, Barbara DeVoe and Robert Kerner recount the stepwise effort they devised to ensure safety in lithotripsy, an example of in-situ simulation in a highly specialized unit. Finally, Kristy Loewenstein in Chapter 13 details her program with highly skilled standardized patients to teach psychiatric personnel how to contend with potentially violent patients in a behavioral health setting, as part of an ambitious initiative to manage aggressive behavior in a humane, patient-focused way.

Finally, we ask readers to take note of the Foreword by Michael J. Dowling, who explains how, in his role as president and chief executive officer of North Shore-LIJ, he developed the concept of a learning organization within a health care system and went on to create the corporate university from which PSI emerged as one of the central components of his visionary commitment to patient safety. His contribution was both foundational and integral to the strategies and processes that we describe throughout this book.

Kathleen Gallo
Lawrence G. Smith

REFERENCES

Christensen, C. M., Anthony, S. D., & Roth, E. A. (2004). *Seeing what's next?: Using the theories of innovation to predict industry change*. Boston, MA: Harvard Business School Press.

Donaldson, L., & Philip, P. (2004). Patient safety: A global priority. *Bull World Health Organ, 82*(12), 892. doi:/S0042-96862004001200002

Dunn, W., Deutsch, E. S., Maxworthy, J., Gallo, K., & Dong, Y. (2013). Systems integration. In A. I. Levine (Ed.), *Comprehensive textbook of healthcare simulation*. New York, NY: Springer Publishing.

Institute of Medicine. (2010). *The future of nursing: Leading change, advancing health*. Washington, DC: National Academies Press.

Kohn, L. T., Corrigan, J., & Donaldson, M. S. (2000). *To err is human: Building a safer health system*. Washington, DC: National Academies Press.

Senge, P. M. (1990). *The fifth discipline:The art and practice of the learning organization* (1st ed.). New York, NY: Doubleday.

Acknowledgments

We personally wish to thank John Galbraith Simmons, the medical writer and author whose contributions, supportive feedback, and writing and editorial skills helped to shape this book from the outset.

We are also ever so grateful to the entire staff at the Center for Learning and Innovation, the Patient Safety Institute, and the Clinical Skills Center. Without their persistent commitment to excellence this story could not have unfolded and could not have been told.

In addition to personal thanks to each of our contributors, who adhered to tight deadlines in spite of imposing schedules, we extend our gratitude to all the North Shore-LIJ clinicians who participate at the Patient Safety Institute. Their outstanding commitment to excellence, interprofessional education, and patient safety helped make this book possible.

Finally, we are most appreciative to Christina Carnesi for her exquisite attention to detail and her ability to organize and coordinate all those on the team who contributed to the completion of this work. We also thank our editors at Springer Publishing Company. Allan Graubard helped us first envision the project and Joseph Morita, the current senior acquisitions editor, provided excellent editorial advice throughout.

We hope that this book will encourage others to use simulation as a platform for interprofessional education in an effort to improve teamwork, communication, and clinical decision making. A positive future for health care tomorrow depends on creating a culture of patient safety today.

One: Call to Action: Improving Patient Safety

Kathleen Gallo
Lawrence G. Smith

Introduction: Patient Safety and Simulation: Present and Future

Patient safety, a constant and timeless goal in medicine, is of paramount concern in an age in which health care delivery, in new and unprecedented ways, demands attention far beyond the ancient imprecation that physicians must "do no harm." As it evolves and matures, engages nurses and physicians at all levels of education and in all capacities, the patient safety movement both strongly embraces an interprofessional model of teamwork and advocates the systematic use of simulation—a multifaceted, multipurpose, and complex tool that we explore throughout this book. Today, its underlying aims in terms of learning, education, and assessment have come together to create a powerful and largely unified set of principles that shape a host of practical applications. The result, broadly speaking, is emergence of a renewed commitment to safety that signals broad, substantive culture change that is already beginning to generate future transformations of the health care landscape (Elwyn & Corrigan, 2005; Small & Barach, 2002).

Principal among the many factors that account for convergence of the patient safety movement and contemporary advances in simulation is the ongoing crisis that affects virtually all health care organizations. Pressing problems include workforce shortages, variations in competence among nurse graduates and physicians alike, and a patient care model that is inconsistent with consumer demand. Allied with these internal issues are various external factors: an aging and diverse population, the exponential expansion of the knowledge base, advances in helpful but potentially harmful technologies, and a consumer movement that demands transparency and participation in patient care and decision making. Add to this the competitive environment that may be expected to persist through implementation of the Affordable Care Act (Oberlander, 2012), whatever its economic and structural consequences, and the result could be described as a perfect storm: a health care system that is unreliable, costly, unsafe, inefficient, and ineffective (Gallo & Smith, 2010; Sanford, 2007; Whitcomb, 2011).

SCOPE AND PURPOSE

Simulation, as we understand and use it and emphasize from the outset, is not a narrow enterprise that aims merely to provide drill systems for training medical personnel or simple "hands-on" learning exercises to reinforce a set of educational objectives (Levine, DeMaria, Schwartz, & Sim, 2013a). Rather, it is an approach that is central to implementing necessary and far-reaching change in the provision of health care.

As we show in Chapter 1, concerning the establishment of the Patient Safety Institute (PSI), simulation can serve as a flexible instrument and conduit for introducing changes in practice and procedures. It is a tool for enhancing teamwork and communication and it can be used to uncover the root causes of medical errors, as a first step in correcting and preventing them. It allows for assessment of individual and team competency, not just recall of facts. It is a reliable process that can be employed on a routine basis in systematic ways; the same basic operational principles and methodology, that is to say, can be used in applying simulation to all disciplines and procedures.

Furthermore, as we discuss more fully below, if it is employed with attention to coherent theoretical and practical bases, simulation can be central to a form of "systems integration" that can positively impact an entire organization (Dunn et al., 2013). The Society for Simulation in Healthcare (SSH) has articulated just such a goal for accrediting programs that "demonstrate consistent, planned, collaborative, integrative and iterative application of simulation-based assessment and teaching activities" with the aim of achieving "excellent bedside clinical care, enhanced patient safety, and improved metrics across the healthcare system" (Deutsch, Mancini, Dunn et al, 2013).

ORIGINS OF THE CONTEMPORARY PATIENT SAFETY MOVEMENT

Current concepts surrounding patient safety percolated through the medical literature during the 1990s and achieved a dramatic breakthrough at the turn of the 21st century with the Institute of Medicine (IOM) publication, *To Err Is Human: Building a Safer Health System* (Kohn, Corrigan, & Donaldson, 2000). Seeking and reaching a broad audience, the 287-page report emerged from the IOM's Committee on Quality of Health Care in America and aimed to initiate long-term improvement in an industry that, by the evidence from a safety standpoint, could only be described as substantially deficient and defective. The dramatic estimate of deaths owing to medical errors, from 44,000 to 98,000 annually, also pointed to a far greater number of preventable medical errors. In addition, *To Err Is Human* drove home the host of negative consequences beyond lost life and unnecessary adverse events: low levels of trust and satisfaction among patients, diminished morale on the part of health care professionals, litigation, and huge financial costs to the system as a whole.

The goal of *To Err Is Human*, however, was not only to bring to light the nature and extent of the problem but "to break this cycle of inaction," and it became an example of how a "policy report can transform a healthcare issue into a national priority" (Stelfox, Palmisani, Scurlock, Orav, & Bates, 2006, p. 177). The IOM also set out a prescriptive and reasoned list of recommendations. Hoping to provide a long-term patient safety strategy, the authors effectively outlined a national agenda: a mandatory error-reporting system, legislation to ensure collection and protection of safety data, higher performance standards, and greater commitment from professional societies and organizations. In addition, the report pointedly advised "Implementing Safety Systems in Health Care Organizations." One among its formal recommendations (8.1) included a set of points worth verbatim citation because they delineate the fundamentals that undergird our efforts at PSI, together with the rationale for its integral status within the North Shore-LIJ Health System. Health care organizations must "develop a culture of safety" and should:

- provide strong, clear and visible attention to safety
- implement nonpunitive systems for reporting and analyzing errors within their organizations
- incorporate well-understood safety principles, such as standardizing and simplifying equipment, supplies, and processes
- establish interdisciplinary team training programs for providers that incorporate proven methods of team training, such as simulation (Kohn et al., 2000, p. 14)

Demonstrating the real-world development and deployment of these notional suggestions constitutes the form and substance of each of the chapters that comprise this book. We should add that today, nearly 15 years after its appearance, as we note in Chapter 3, *To Err Is Human* has impacted the patient safety movement in ways comparable to Abraham Flexner's 1910 report advocating changes that, a century ago, were imperative to impose if the American medical establishment were to embrace the advent of scientific medicine (Cooke, Irby, Sullivan, & Ludmerer, 2006). Today in health care, the exponential expansion of the knowledge base and new information streams require nothing less with respect to patient safety.

TEAMWORK TRUMPS AUTONOMY

Simulation, as we understand and use it, is an eminently interprofessional endeavor. Both historically and conceptually, recognizing the value added by teams comprised of physicians, nurses, and other providers working together has been crucial to organizing the use of simulation. Vast shifts in the medical marketplace in the final decades of the 20th century brought into question the control that the "medical profession"—headed by physicians—could wield over "markets, organizations, and standards of judgment"(Starr & American Council of Learned Societies, 1982, p. 421). Far-reaching advances in treating and managing many previously unrecognized and untreatable diseases generated not only institutional change and economic transformations but also raised many of the serious safety issues that undermined the concept of the doctor-in-charge as the autonomous decision maker. Although the "hierarchy gradient" remains a legacy issue in need of attention and resolution, there is today widespread acknowledgment that the safety net in medicine must be the team and not the individual (Thistlethwaite, Moran, and World Health Organization Study Group on Interprofessional Education and Collaborative Practice, 2010).

It is teams working together that enable more complex tasks to be accomplished safely, competently, and effectively—and, in fact, there would be little point to simulation as we employ it, without them. The platforms we develop in simulation are important not only "for the acquisition of critical skills in each of the [health] professions, but they can also be a powerful means for teaching and assessing team-based competencies interprofessionally" (Thibault, 2013, p. 1931). "Teamwork trumps autonomy" is not a slogan but an imperative.

ADVANCING A NEW PARADIGM

Both conceptually and historically, simulation for patient safety owes much to measures first developed in industries outside health care. Aviation is the field most directly responsible. Although the use of "flight simulators" to train pilots and crew dates to the first decades of the 20th century, the principles of crew resource management (CRM), so crucial to airline safety, developed over a quarter of a century beginning in the 1970s (Helmreich, 2000). They included attention to human interaction, an emphasis on team-based cooperation, and a "shift away from autocratic and individualistic styles of aircraft command" to one that is "team based with mutual interdependence and shared responsibility"(Musson & Helmreich, 2004, p. 26). In addition, the founders of CRM created the basic format of extensive postincident, nondidactic, nonhierarchical debriefings that are carried out in conjunction with every high-fidelity flight simulation.

Adaptation of CRM techniques to medicine occurred first in anesthesiology, closely associated with pioneering explorations by David Gaba at Stanford University. He and colleagues developed Anesthesiology Crisis Resource Management (ACRM) in the late 1980s. They used an off-the-shelf manikin, re-engineered for computerized simulation of several physiologic variables, including electrocardiogram (ECG), heart rate, blood pressure, and oximetry. Teams were interprofessional, comprised of nurses and an operating surgeon in addition to the anesthesiologist. The first course in ACRM, in 1990, included most if not all the elements that would go on to define medical simulation today: pre-assigned reading, brief scenarios to emulate critical events, video recording of sessions, and facilitated debriefings based on the aviation industry model (Gaba, Fish, Smith & Sowb, 2001).

Use of simulation may focus on patient safety but, it should be added, its broader potential has always been understood: It is a tool for education and assessment. In an independent and parallel development, also working in anesthesia, Michael Good and colleagues at the University of Florida at Gainesville developed a manikin simulation program that they used to teach basic procedures and techniques. Their efforts, also beginning in the 1980s, evolved into several extensive projects to create computer-controlled simulators that could be manufactured and marketed commercially. The Gainesville group represented one of a number of successful efforts to advance manikin technology in ways to enhance fidelity during simulation (Rosen, 2013).

Anesthesiology, as a surgery-related specialty that requires teamwork by definition, was a logical domain to present the case for simulation, and it turned into a gateway for other domains and specialties. As Gaba enumerated them in 2001, not long after publication of *To Err Is Human*, the first of these included the intensive care unit, emergency medicine bays, and the specialties of cardiology, radiology, and obstetrics (Gaba, 2001). Subsequent research concerning the efficacy and effectiveness of simulation, as expected, proved to be a difficult proposition—it is still a work-in-progress—and a dearth of head-to-head studies may have slowed its widespread adoption. But it remains that today, within a short span of 2 decades, "healthcare simulation has gone from 'best secret' to 'best practice'" (Levine et al., 2013a, p. 4).

HOW IT'S DONE: TYPES AND MODALITIES

Simulation is employed to educate trainees, providing advanced learning to experienced providers, and for assessment at all levels. While use of the manikin has been the most prominent modality and may be considered the "mainstay of simulation training" (Hope & Chin, 2008, p. 82), it should be understood in context. Today there are dozens of models—partial and full-sized, neonatal, pediatric, and adult; yet they are best viewed not as indispensable technologies but as fundamentally useful props. In guided learning contexts and with the help of debriefing, they can be put to a multitude of uses. High-fidelity simulation generally refers to the computer-based applications for which the manikin is programmed and, if it possesses interactive capabilities, it can evince signs and symptoms and react to various stimuli and interventions. Representing a further advance, the so-called haptic devices incorporate tactile feedback technology and have found a growing number of applications. Remote interactions, including the patient's voice and symptoms such as wheezing or coughing, are generally initiated during simulation scenarios from the observation booth.

The "standardized patient" (SP) or "confederate"—the human actor who portrays a patient, family member, or physician—is equally important to simulation. Originating in the 1960s, for many years SPs found employment in assessment, frequently as part of the objective structured clinical exam (OSCE; Wallace, 1997). They play a wider role in simulation today, research supports their use, and they can be employed in conjunction with high-fidelity manikins and in scenarios that aim at improving communications skills, such as delivery of bad news and discussions of adverse events (Howley, 2013). A key advantage to the use of SPs, whether alone or in such hybrid contexts, is their participation in post-simulation assessments and debriefs, where they provide useful emotional feedback to learners. In developing PSI, which today serves both experienced health care providers, new employees, and medical students, we inaugurated a Clinical Skills Center that trains and deploys SPs in any number of venues.

All these modalities are discussed in the various chapters in this book. At PSI we put the various models of computerized manikins to a range of uses, sometimes in combination with SPs. Our endovascular simulator,[1] a haptic device, is principally employed to train cardiac fellows but may be adapted for use with other specialties such as neurosurgery and vascular surgery. Our de-escalation program in behavioral health uses standardized patients exclusively, with actors trained to portray patients in acute states of decompensation; they are similarly engaged to help improve communications skills in both pediatrics and cardiology. We use both the manikin and standardized patients in behavioral health emergencies and in all programs for emergency-related pediatrics.

ASPECTS OF ADULT LEARNING

Whatever modality employed, simulation is a form of adult learning. Its principles, as they have developed over the past 3 decades, pay tribute to classical theories that emphasize the singular ways in which adults learn, the crucial importance of experiential learning (Kolb, 1984), and investigations into the most effective ways that professionals act, or "reflection-in-action" (Schön, 1983). Adults bring knowledge to learning situations; they are goal- and relevancy-oriented, self-directed, and favor practical aims (Knowles, 1980). These theories all align with and favor teamwork and interprofessional learning in health care (Oandasan & Reeves, 2005). Two concepts stand out across all modes of simulation for patient safety: debriefing and deliberate practice.

Deliberate practice has proved to be a crucial organizing concept. It expresses revision of the widely held view that individuals differ greatly in their potential for acquiring various skills, and that they reach an asymptotic limit beyond which they cannot improve. Emerging from empirical research by cognitive scientist K. Anders Ericsson and based on information processing theory, deliberate practice points to two key features of simulation that are requisite for success: repetition and guided practice (Ericsson, 1993). Deliberate practice has been described as "an important property of powerful [simulation-based medical] interventions used to shape, refine, and maintain trainee knowledge, skills and attitudes" (McGaghie, Issenberg, Petrusa, & Scalese, 2010, p. 55).

Extensive debriefing is so crucial to interprofessional simulation that without it, the activity might best be described as of no value. The postsimulation debriefing is not a short discussion but typically lasts longer than the simulation scenario itself. Closely examined in terms of concepts that derive from educational theory (Lederman, 1992), the fundamental principles of nonthreatening, facilitated debriefing, as noted above and as we describe and discuss them in Chapter 2, originated with CRM. From the Center for Medical Simulation (CMS) at Harvard Medical School there has since emerged the cluster of concepts known as "Debriefing with Good Judgment" that rationalizes and refines the process for simulation in health care (Rudolph, Simon, Dufresne, & Raemer, 2006). This stepwise approach incorporates the theory of reflective practice with emphasis on learners' assumptions, their "mental frameworks," and a form of guided facilitation, known as "advocacy-inquiry," which enables identification and remediation of knowledge and performance gaps.

THE BIGGER PICTURE: SIMULATION, HEALTH CARE, AND SYSTEMS INTEGRATION

Simulation for patient safety, as it has evolved over the past 15 years, has proved to be just as rich in theory as it is extensive in range of application (Bradley, 2006). When employed effectively, it represents a form of systems engineering (SE) used to address one of the most pressing problems in health care, with the elaboration of qualitative and quantitative concepts and methodologies suited to creating and improving systems that are effective, efficient, and patient-centered (*Building a Better Delivery System: A New Engineering/Health Care Partnership*, 2005). From a design and engineering perspective, health care organizations are *complex adaptive systems* (Rouse, 2008). That is to say that they are dynamic and technologically complex, comprised of multiple components and populated by a variety of agents and stakeholders; they are also subject to external forces, such as regulatory agencies and market forces, and are neither predictable nor steady-state. Above all, such systems benefit from quality-improvement strategies and methods, such as Six Sigma and Lean, and constitute a comprehensive engineering toolkit. In this context, simulation and the interprofessional learning model represent a combined educational matrix, both of them disruptive innovations in health care that aim to build an organizational culture of safety.

Our initiative in perinatal services, discussed at length in Chapter 7, can serve as a brief real-world illustration of process and application.[2] In 2008, prompted by adverse events, clinical service and risk management personnel, together with PSI leadership, collaborated to provide a root cause analysis using both process and SE tools such as flowcharting and statistical process control. Results enabled the integrated development of a comprehensive safety initiative comprised of formalized interprofessional team training, renewed emphasis on communication, assessment of competence in electronic fetal monitoring, and simulation for high-risk obstetrics emergency procedures together with a targeted educational curriculum. A research component built into the initiative enabled validation (Wagner et al., 2012).

Simulation used in this way, to perform analysis and implement changes to improve patient safety, constitutes the strategy and process of systems integration (SI) in a health care system. The SSH recognizes SI as an accreditation standard for programs that employ simulation in ways consonant with goals and principles set out by the IOM's canonical reports.[3] Although "integration" and "continuum of care" have been concepts in health care for a generation, simulation today represents a practical tool for designing and putting to use solutions based on sound and tested principles of process and SE.

FUTURE DIFFUSION

Pondering the future in 2004, David Gaba identified no less than ten "driving forces and implementation mechanisms" by which simulation—and, by extension, teamwork and interprofessional education—might be integrated into the fabric of health care (Gaba, 2004, Table 1, p. i8). In addition to simulation societies and research teams, stakeholders would include health care systems, educational institutions and professional societies, the accrediting organizations such as the Accreditation Council for Graduate Medical Education (ACGME), various funders and nongovernmental organizations, the concerned public, and government policy entities. Speculating on what might come to pass, Gaba imagined two contrasting futures: one in which, by 2025, simulation was extensively used and fully accepted, and another, more pessimistic outcome, in which it failed to live up to its potential and could not win enough support to sustain continued adoption. He suggested that simulation was close to a threshold of tipping point or threshold for "a revolutionary change in health care" that would be evident by 2014 though it would take another decade to fully evolve (Gaba, 2004, p. i9).

Today, at that 10-year midway point in time, simulation is indeed moving toward widespread adoption and full-scale diffusion. Disruptive innovations always entail early adopters, late adopters, and a cautious broad middle; subsequent diffusion after development of a critical mass is a long and nonrigid process of adaptation (Rogers, 2004) . But the "vision of simulation embedded in the fabric of care" (Gaba, 2004, p. i7) is on its way to becoming a ubiquitous reality for learning and assessment alike (Levine et al., 2013b). With respect to its potential, we should add that the interprofessional model and the imperative to reduce preventable harm have created innumerable rich contexts for further innovation, for research into all the interactive and cognitive components that underlie adult learning, and for investigations and initiatives that advance the broader goal of building a robust culture of patient safety. Each of the chapters in this book represents a further step along that path.

NOTES

1. Simantha®: Medical Simulation Corporation.
2. For further examples of the strategic application of SE processes, see also Chapter 3 (sepsis) and Chapter 11 (critical care nurse fellowship program).
3. In addition to *To Err Is Human* (Kohn et al., 2000), these include *Crossing the Quality Chasm* (2001), *Envisioning the National Health Care Quality Report* (2001), *Priority Areas for National Action* (2003), and other publications.

REFERENCES

Bradley, P. (2006). The history of simulation in medical education and possible future directions. *Medical Education, 40*(3), 254–262. doi:10.1111/j.1365-2929.2006.02394.x

Building a better delivery system: A new engineering/health care partnership. (2005). Washington, DC: The National Academies Press.

Cooke, M., Irby, D. M., Sullivan, W., & Ludmerer, K. M. (2006). American medical education 100 years after the Flexner report. *The New England Journal of Medicine, 355*(13), 1339–1344. doi:10.1056/NEJMra055445

Deutsch, E. S., Mancini, M. B., Dunn, W. F., et al. (2013). Informational guide for the accreditation process. http://www.ssih.org/Accreditation/Full-Accreditation. Accessed June 28, 2014.

Dunn, W. D. E., Maxworthy. J., Gallo. K., Dong, Y., Manos, J., Pendergrass, T., & Brazil, V. (2013). Systems integration. In A. I. Levine, S. DeMaria, Jr., A. D. Schwartz, & A. J. Sim (Ed.), *The comprehensive textbook of healthcare simulation* (pp. 95–110). New York, NY: Springer.

Elwyn, G., & Corrigan, J. M. (2005). The patient safety story. *BMJ, 331*(7512), 302–304. doi:10.1136/bmj.38562.690104.43

Ericsson, K. A. (1993). The role of deliberate practice in the acquisition of expert performance. *Psychological Review, 100*(3), 363–406.

Gaba, D. M. (2004). The future vision of simulation in health care. *Quality & Safety in Health Care, 13*(Suppl. 1), i2–i10. doi:10.1136/qhc.13.suppl_1.i2

Gaba, D. M, H. S., Fish, K. J., Smith, B. E., Sowb, Y. A. (2001). Simulation-based training in anesthesia crisis resource management (ACRM): A decade of experience. *Simulation and Gaming, 32*(2), 175–193.

Gallo, K., & Smith, L. (2010). Meeting tomorrow's health care needs: Teamwork trumps autonomy. *Nursing Education Perspectives, 31*(4), 207.

Helmreich, R. L. (2000). On error management: Lessons from aviation. *BMJ, 320*(7237), 781–785.

Hope, G., & Chin, C. (2008). Equipment. In R. H. Riley (Ed.), *Manual of simulation in healthcare* (pp. 81–86). New York, NY: Oxford.

Howley, L. (2013). Standardized patients. In A. I. Levine, S. Demaria, Jr., A. D. Schwartz, & A. J. Sim (Ed.), *The comprehensive textbook of healthcare simulation*. New York, NY: Springer.

Institute of Medicine (2001). *Crossing the quality chasm: A new health system for the 21st century*. Washington, DC: National Academy Press.

Knowles, M. S. (1980). *The modern practice of adult education: From pedagogy to andragogy* (Rev. and updated ed.). New York, NY: Cambridge, The Adult Education.

Kohn, L. T., Corrigan, J., & Donaldson, M. S. (2000). *To err is human: Building a safer health system*. Washington, DC: National Academy Press.

Kolb, D. A. (1984). *Experiential learning: Experience as the source of learning and development*. Englewood Cliffs, NJ: Prentice-Hall.

Lederman, L. (1992). Debriefing: Toward a systematic assessment of theory and practice. *Simulation and Gaming, 23*(2), 145–160.

Levine, A. I., DeMaria, S. Jr., Schwartz, A. D., & Sim, A. J. (2013a). Healthcare simulation: From 'Best Secret' to 'Best Practice'. In A. I. Levine, S. DeMaria, Jr., A. D. Schwartz, & A. J. Sim (Ed.), *The comprehensive textbook of healthcare simulation*. New York, NY: Springer.

Levine, A. I., DeMaria, S. Jr., Schwartz, A. D., & Sim, A. J. (2013b). A Future Vision. In A. I. Levine, S. DeMaria, Jr., A. D. Schwartz, & A. J. Sim (Ed.), *The comprehensive textbook of healthcare simulation* (pp. 649–653). New York, NY: Springer.

McGaghie, W. C., Issenberg, S. B., Petrusa, E. R., & Scalese, R. J. (2010). A critical review of simulation-based medical education research: 2003–2009. *Medical Education, 44*(1), 50–63. doi:10.1111/j.1365-2923.2009.03547.x

Musson, D., & Helmreich, R. (2004). Team training and resource management in healthcare: Current issues and future directions. *Harvard Health Policy Review, 5*(1), 25–35.

National Center for Interprofessiona Practice and Education. Retrieved from http://nexusipe.org/about

Oandasan, I., & Reeves, S. (2005). Key elements of interprofessional education. Part 2: Factors, processes and outcomes. *Journal of Interprofessional Care, 19*(Suppl. 1), 39–48. doi:10.1080/13561820500 081703

Oberlander, J. (2012). The future of obamacare. *The New England Journal of Medicine, 367*(23), 2165–2167. doi:10.1056/NEJMp1213674

Priority Areas for National Action: Transforming Health Care Quality. (2003). The National Academies Press.

Rogers, E. M. (2004). A prospective and retrospective look at the diffusion model. *Journal of Health Communication, 9*(Suppl. 1), 13–19. doi:10.1080/10810730490271449

Rosen, K. (2013). History of simulation. In A. I. Levine, S. DeMaria, Jr., A. D. Schwartz, & A. J. Sim (Ed.), *The comprehensive textbook of healthcare simulation* (pp. 5–49). New York, NY: Springer.

Rouse, W. (2008). Health care as a complex adaptive system: Implications for design and management. *The Bridge, 38*(1), 17–24.

Rudolph, J. W., Simon, R., Dufresne, R. L., & Raemer, D. B. (2006). There's no such thing as "nonjudgmental" debriefing: A theory and method for debriefing with good judgment. *Simulation in Healthcare, 1*(1), 49–55.

Sanford, K. (2007). Confronting the perfect storm: A challenge to nurse leaders. *Nursing Administration Quarterly, 31*(2), 120–123. doi:10.1097/01.NAQ.0000264859.64464.af

Schön, D. A. (1983). *The reflective practitioner: How professionals think in action.* New York, NY: Basic Books.

Small, S. D., & Barach, P. (2002). Patient safety and health policy: A history and review. *Hematology Oncology Clinics of North America, 16*(6), 1463–1482.

Starr, P., & American Council of Learned Societies. (1982). *The social transformation of American medicine* (pp. xiv, 514 p.). Retrieved from http://www.columbia.edu/cgi-bin/cul/resolve?clio8861872

Stelfox, H. T., Palmisani, S., Scurlock, C., Orav, E. J., & Bates, D. W. (2006). The "To err is human" report and the patient safety literature. *Quality & Safety in Health Care, 15*(3), 174–178. doi:10.1136/qshc.2006.017947

Thibault, G. E. (2013). Reforming health professions education will require culture change and closer ties between classroom and practice. *Health Affairs (Millwood), 32*(11), 1928–1932. doi:10.1377/hlthaff.2013.0827

Thistlethwaite, J., Moran, M., World Health Organization Study Group on Interprofessional Education and Collaborative Practice. (2010). Learning outcomes for interprofessional education (IPE): Literature review and synthesis. *Journal of Interprofessional Care, 24*(5), 503–513. doi:10.3109/13561820.2010.483366

Wagner, B., Meirowitz, N., Shah, J., Nanda, D., Reggio, L., Cohen, P., Britt, K., . . . Abrams, K. J. (2012). Comprehensive perinatal safety initiative to reduce adverse obstetric events. *Journal of Healthcare Quality, 34*(1), 6–15. doi:10.1111/j.1945-1474.2011.00134.x

Wallace, P. (1997). Following the threads of an innovation: The history of standardized patients in medical education. *Caduceus, 13*(2), 5–28.

Whitcomb, M. E. (2011). Commentary: Meeting future medical care needs: A perfect storm on the horizon. *Academic Medicine, 86*(12), 1490–1491. doi:10.1097/ACM.0b013e318235d5d4

John Galbraith Simmons

1: Launching PSI: Establishing a Culture of Patient Safety

The Patient Safety Institute (PSI), one of the most extensive simulation centers currently in operation, provides a safe environment for collaborative educational experiences in which learners can acquire and improve clinical skills, critical thinking abilities, and the capacity to work in teams. Designed in accordance with principles of adult education and deliberate practice, the PSI plays a strategic role within a broader educational context in the second largest nonprofit, secular health care system in the country.

DEVELOPING A LEARNING ORGANIZATION

Founding and organizing the PSI represented not so much the gradual evolution of an idea but, rather, the concrete result and practical outcome of broad organizational aspirations. In 2001 Michael Dowling, then executive vice president of the North Shore-LIJ (NS-LIJ), soon to become its chief operating officer, prepared a white paper in which he proposed establishing a "leadership institute" to facilitate a culture of continuous learning among all its employees (Dowling, 2001). While concern for quality of personnel was nothing new, Dowling faced a major task in forging a unified culture in a large, newly formed health care system comprised of two recently merged metropolitan hospitals and a growing number of small community hospitals and ambulatory services. The broader historic context was the "emergence of large-scale systems" in health care in the United States, an institutional transformation in that field unrivaled in magnitude since creation of the modern hospital system in the late 19th century (Stevens, 1989).

Dowling was disposed by his background in both administration and education to observe that "performance management" was "one of the least developed areas" in health care (Dowling, 2001). With a master's degree in social work, he had entered the field of corporate health care after serving as New York State's director of Health, Education and Human Services for 7 years and as commissioner of the state's Department of Social Services; he had also taught at Fordham University Graduate School of Social Services, where he was assistant dean and professor of social policy. His proposal to create a leadership institute bore the overall aim of turning it into a "learning organization" whose employees could help it adapt to the changing "consumer-focused competitive landscape." This broad idea encountered some resistance among other executives but the pressing need for a workforce with a shared identity and values in one of the largest integrated health systems in the United States, newly born of mergers and acquisitions, worked in his favor. The Center for Learning and Innovation (CLI) opened in 2002, the same year Dowling was named CEO of the entire organization.

CLI—from which PSI would soon emerge—was designed as a "corporate university," the first such entity established within a health care system, and it would eventually become the largest of its kind in the United States. Historically, learning facilities operating under a corporate umbrella with strategic aims date to the 1950s, and Dowling had spent time at GE Crotonville, which General Electric had established in 1956 (Assen, 2010; GE Crotonville, n.d.). Both General Electric and the Harvard School of Public Health, recruited as strategic partners, helped design CLI; its name, incidentally, originated with NS-LIJ health system employees.

Patient safety as an institutional aim at CLI would represent a logical but not self-evident shift in focus after the corporate university took steps to cultivate the workforce through education and to regard its members as a resource for innovation, efficiency, and improvement (Gebauer, Lowman, & Gordon, 2008). As chief learning officer (CLO), Dowling appointed Kathleen Gallo; and soon after, as a strategic decision, he asked her to also manage human resources (HR) for the entire system. With a doctorate in nursing, a background in trauma care and emergency medicine, and a degree in business administration, Gallo was aware, like Dowling, of the advantages that might be had by applying lessons from industries outside health care (Chassin, 2013). She viewed the founding of CLI as a form of disruptive innovation in health care that would generate a new pedagogical model. She helped design and implement CLI's entire program, which offered courses for managers and executives, and she instituted "Six Sigma," the quality assurance and efficiency system closely associated with GE. She also implemented a leader-as-teacher model whereby executive leadership partnered with the CLI team and became faculty for the management programs. In her dual role, she spent the best part of 4 years integrating recruitment, personnel functions, and learning activities across the entire organization.

But as an academic and, unlike most HR executives, also trained as a nurse, Gallo's instinct was always to return to clinical issues. The most pressing of these to emerge in health care, coincidentally with the founding of CLI, was patient safety.

IMPACT OF *TO ERR IS HUMAN*

In terms of raising awareness, *To Err Is Human*, the Institute of Medicine (IOM) report published in late 1999, had a seismic impact on medicine in the United States (Kohn, Corrigan, & Donaldson, 2000). Its system-wide scope—the 287-page report did not focus on physicians or exclusively on hospitals but covered the whole realm of health care delivery—sent a powerful message: The industry was not safe and most errors were preventable. Medical missteps that resulted in death—as many as 98,000 annually—constituted only the tip of the error iceberg. The report won widespread attention in the media and in Congress, and it stimulated a variety of governmental and organizational initiatives (Stelfox, Palmisani, Scurlock, Orav, & Bates, 2006), including establishment of a database by the Agency for Healthcare Research and Quality and attention from (as it's now known) The Joint Commission (Blouin & McDonagh, 2011).

Importantly, *To Err Is Human*, as the title indicated, was not devoted to exposé and blame. It dispensed with the older tendency to examine error in terms of egregious mistakes, incompetent clinicians, or dysfunctional institutions. Instead it focused on human factors, the failures of people to work together in teams, and the lack of a culture of safety. The IOM report straightforwardly estimated the cost of preventable errors at from $38 to $50 billion annually. It also contained two broad recommendations that directly aligned with Michael Dowling's vision of a continuous learning experience and with Gallo's charge as CLO. These were, first, to "make patient safety a priority corporate objective" (p. 166) and, in addition, to "create a learning environment" (p. 178) (Kohn et al., 2000).

SAFETY AND SIMULATION

Off the printed page, Kathleen Gallo had the first glimmer of how patient safety might have an integral fit with CLI in 2004 when, at a national conference for CLOs, she met Michael Barger. He was the CLO of Jet Blue, the airline he had helped found in 1999, and a former TOPGUN in the U.S. Navy, with experience training fighter pilots. With a doctorate in education, Barger headed the airline's own corporate university counterpart to CLI. He effectively introduced Gallo to the widespread use of simulation for safety in the airline industry, lending substance to ideas that she had read about in the IOM report but had not otherwise encountered. Barger explained in some detail how pilots and flight crews trained in teams and used constructed scenarios to prevent disaster. The airline industry, well-known as a model for safety, extensively employed simulation not only to train but to augment teamwork. A learning instrument and an assessment platform at once, it prepared crews for the rare but catastrophic events that cause planes to crash.

Gallo was intrigued by the possibilities for simulation, with which she was not familiar beyond the bare recommendations of the IOM report. The idea seemed attractive: "to be able to deconstruct any adverse event that occurred in the hospital with clinical teams, so that we could learn exactly what happened, and then put together a program that would redesign clinical care to prevent the error from occurring again." Although simulation for teaching in modern medicine was not new, it was limited—a minor aspect of medical and nursing education. If one meant using a puppet-like "phantom" to help learn forceps delivery or practicing hypodermic injection on a tennis ball, simulation was quite old (Gardner & Raemer, 2008). Life-size blue-suited Resusci Annie, the manikin for cardiopulmonary resuscitation that dated to 1960, was a "task trainer"; so were computer-based software packages marketed beginning in the 1980s (Rosen, 2008). In addition, medical schools employed live "standardized patients," mostly for performance assessment (Wallace, 1997).

But simulation that aimed specifically at improving patient safety and teamwork was a more recent development. In only one specialty, anesthesiology, was high-fidelity, or computer-assisted, simulation already well advanced (Gaba, Howard, Fish, Smith, & Sowb, 2001). Success in that field, initially motivated by concern over rising malpractice insurance costs and spearheaded by David Gaba at the Stanford University School of Medicine, helped stoke interest in other fields and was no longer confined to a few institutions. But implementation was for the most part still spotty, theoretical, and, in spite of growing efforts of several fledgling groups, largely unorganized. In terms of scale, simulation as a way to create a culture of safety within a large health care system was almost as uncommon in 2004 as it had been at the tail end of 1999, when *To Err Is Human* was first published (Leape & Berwick, 2005). As Jeffrey B. Cooper, a proponent and professor of anesthesiology, noted at the time: "Simulation in healthcare education and training appears to be gaining acceptance, but it has not yet reached what would be called a 'tipping point' of widespread adoption" (Cooper & Taqueti, 2004, p. i16). Although the authors of the IOM report recommended the use of simulation "whenever possible," it was only one among a welter of policy suggestions to emerge from that document. Few readers would then have heard of crew resource management (CRM), which the report also mentioned.

"Building a culture of safety is proving to be an immense task," wrote Lucian Leape and Donald Berwick 5 years later, in 2005. Both had served on the committee that produced the IOM report: "[A]nd the barriers are formidable. Whether significant progress will be achieved in the next 5 years depends on how successfully those barriers are addressed" (Leape & Berwick, 2005, p. 2385). Progress, they noted, was "frustratingly slow." At the same time, a culture of safety was an aspiration consistent with the breadth of vision that Dowling had articulated in proposing the learning institute that became CLI. Gallo, turning to clinical issues after years spent organizing CLI's management and leadership programs at NS-LIJ, recognized its broad, system-wide potential.

MISSION: CONCEPTION AND ALIGNMENT

Gallo soon learned more. Mike Barger was aware of the first academic efforts to adapt CRM principles to health care. He put her in touch with Robert L.

Helmreich and later in 2004 she traveled to Austin, Texas, to meet him. A professor of psychology—he died in 2012—Helmreich had worked on airline safety and was one of the original architects of CRM. He focused on human factors and his work was strongly data-driven. He had made detailed studies of a large number of airline accidents and disasters; then, after publishing extensively on aviation-related safety and spaceflight (he also worked with NASA and analyzed the behavior of astronauts), he turned to medicine. There his research tracked safety in the operating room and he had followed the same pattern, recording actual procedures and developing a typology of the communications breakdowns that led to preventable surgical errors. In 2000, when *To Err Is Human* was published, he had summarized his research in an article in the *British Medical Journal*. With respect to simulation, he wrote pointedly that "such [simulation] training needs to be ongoing, because in the absence of recurrent training and reinforcement, attitudes and practices decay; and secondly, it needs to be tailored to conditions and experience within organizations" (Helmreich, 2000, p. 783)

With gathering conviction that patient safety both deserved institutional support and had a good fit with CLI, Gallo pursued the literature, learning about Gaba's work, for example, but also more broadly about the educational philosophy underlying adult learning. She had herself been taught in a nursing silo and recognized that classroom experience had a poor fit with the team approach that was more typical in her field of emergency medicine, which was a relatively new specialty (Zink, 2006). About the same time, in early 2005 she also visited the Peter M. Winter Institute for Simulation Education and Research (WISER) at the University of Pittsburgh School of Medicine. Here she saw firsthand the current high-fidelity manikins and could begin to contemplate what a stand-alone institute might accomplish. A decade earlier, anesthesiologist Peter Winter had developed a small simulation suite and some of the medical school faculty over the next several years added curricula and broadened its scope. Established in 2001, WISER had contributed to the development of SimMan® (Laerdal), and 2 years later it opened as the largest dedicated simulation center in the United States (Peter, n.d.).

Gallo returned from Pittsburgh convinced that simulation might work for CLI; it would be an undertaking consistent with the corporate university's overall mission. An additional factor, underscoring the importance of clinical education, was publication of a second IOM report in 2003, *Health Professions Education: A Bridge to Quality.* That document emphasized the need for a substantial shift in educational strategy and methodology, replacing the older model of professional autonomy with one that emphasized teamwork and interprofessional learning. The aim, to improve safety, was in full alignment with the theory underlying clinical simulation (Institute of Medicine, 2003; Jeffries, 2009). Gallo recognized that the literature brought up a number of concepts that comported readily with the aims of the "profound culture change" that Dowling had forecast in 2001. The new pursuit of patient safety through the rationalized use of simulation could indeed be, if properly mounted, an instance of disruptive innovation applied to health care (Bower & Christensen, 1995).

To be sure, in terms of the real world, the evidence base in terms of producing safety through the guided use of simulation was yet to create a wellspring of enthusiasm; but a Best Evidence Medical Education (BEME) review in 2005, for which the lead author was high-fidelity simulation expert S. Barry Issenberg, was highly encouraging (Issenberg, McGaghie, Petrusa, Lee Gordon, & Scalese, 2005). Even without a surfeit of evidence, simulation was eminently worth a try. As Gaba and others often pointed out, the airline industry did not and could scarcely be expected to use randomized trials before adopting CRM (Rosen, 2008). As he noted in a paper published in 2004, "Pioneering centres in health care are starting to take the leap of long-term application with less than absolute proof of benefit" (Gaba, 2004, p. i7).

Gallo talked with Dowling about the prospect of a pilot project and he agreed. In 2005 they set aside a small budget. At Glen Cove Hospital, two labor and delivery rooms were identified as available and could serve for space; Gallo hired a staff of one—Barbara DeVoe, as CLI's director of clinical education.

PSI: ESTABLISHMENT AND FIRST STEPS

So in late June 2005, DeVoe watched with concentrated attention as a sales representative put together the various parts of the Laerdal manikin known as SimMan, which had been delivered in boxes to the Center for Learning and Innovation. She was charged with and intent upon learning everything that the full-sized computer-driven manikin could do. Trained, like Gallo, in emergency medicine, DeVoe had also worked as a critical care nurse and nurse practitioner before moving into administration. Now she paid attention as the manikin was fitted and bolted together from the tip of his toes to the top of his head and connected to the computer feedback system. Soon after, Dowling and other executives came out to the hospital as she demonstrated some of its capabilities and responses to computer-controlled inputs.

The first year at the small, still unnamed institute in Glen Cove was given over to proof of concept and, as it turned out, to first steps in aligning theory and practice. Although there were more lethal preventable errors, as *To Err Is Human* reported, than deaths from motor vehicle accidents, AIDS, or breast cancer, the numbers were invisible in individual departmental metrics (Naik & Brien, 2013). Without a statistical blunt weapon, the problem of effectively organizing high fidelity simulation for patient safety that was not narrowly focused on task training was twofold. First, who from the hospital would serve as interested stakeholders? And second, how was simulation to work in actual practice? What would it look like (Kerner, 2010)?

Gallo found a solution to this start-up issue by making use of the health system's new Critical Care Nurse Fellowship Program (CCNFP), just initiated at North Shore-LIJ in 2005 (Friedman, Cooper, Click, & Fitzpatrick, 2011; Friedman, Delaney, Schmidt, Quinn, & Macyk, 2013) (see Chapter 11). Owing to stress and burnout, retention rates for new nurse graduates in acute care settings were known to be low; in metropolitan New York they were alarmingly so. The CCNFP proposed to remedy high attrition by offering new nurses a critical care core curriculum, seminars, and assigned preceptors, among other components. Some 30 nurses would work through the program each year. Into this blended learning platform Gallo introduced a simulation program. Nurses ran through a gamut of emergency and critical care procedures, with scenarios crafted in line with the curriculum they followed. They reported greater comfort and confidence when actually deployed to clinical units. Research would show the program to be both cost saving and successful in its aim to retain nurses; it has expanded to include other subdisciplines and continues to the present.

Despite the nurses' promising reception of simulation, the physical setup at Glen Cove proved inadequate. Barbara DeVoe worked the manikin during scenarios while seated at the computer; she served as its voice and worked the controls. But she and a colleague would be in the same room with the nurses and they tended to notice; instead of paying attention to the manikin, they would look at her. After calling each session, she would also run debriefings—fairly informal discussions at first. "It was totally unrealistic," DeVoe recalls. As the language of simulation would later put it, if psychological fidelity could be described as passable, physical and environmental fidelity were lacking.

FRAMEWORK: DEFINED AND EXPANDED

Within a year from its beginnings at Glen Cove, PSI was formally named and established at a 5,000 square-foot facility at NS-LIJ in Hauppauge, Long Island New York, with Barbara DeVoe promoted as director. Here the physical design was in line with the more advanced simulation centers that were beginning to crop up elsewhere in the United States. Gallo and DeVoe had visited several of the major ones: the Simulation Center at Hartford Hospital in Connecticut; the Gordon Center at the University of Miami Miller School of Medicine (where the Harvey® high-fidelity manikin had been developed); and the Center for Experiential Learning & Assessment at Vanderbilt University. The PSI incorporated the common elements of design: control rooms with one-way mirrors that looked onto clinical and procedure rooms, an emergency disaster suite, and an operating room. There was a separate classroom and, to transport learners to the center from the health system hospitals, the institute purchased a bus.

In and of itself, the move to a larger, state-of-the-art facility did not reflect a more profound development in the intellectual framework. At the beginning, the technology of the operation seemed impressive. High-fidelity simulators such as SimMan, followed by still more sophisticated models, made use of impressive technologies to simulate a variety of conditions for learning exercises. They impressed students, nurses, and physicians alike. Gradually—others have described the same learning curve—Gallo and DeVoe came to realize that the high-fidelity manikin was a means to an end; it was essentially a prop (Kerner, 2010; Lampotang, 2008). If it were to become genuinely effective, simulation required the underpinnings of an educational philosophy that was beginning, in the wake of such publications as *To Err Is Human*, to promise genuine impact on health care delivery and patient safety. "It had started out being about the technology and all the tasks you could do," remembered DeVoe, "but as time went on we came to the realization that it was far more than technology." Gallo and DeVoe discovered or rediscovered it for themselves and this view—that successful use of simulation in medicine was not at root beholden to technology but represented an educational philosophy in action in which interprofessional learning was critical—became widely shared in the field (Society for Simulation in Healthcare, 2013).

If developed in line with recommendations in the 2003 IOM report, *Health Professions Education*, PSI would help health care providers in all capacities deliver patient-centered care rooted in evidence-based medicine, and it would emphasize team training. But a deeper look into the research that supported the IOM recommendation led directly to educational concepts that could be used in concrete ways to design simulation, carry out scenarios, and assess performance. Simulation raised the larger question of mastery, in fact, in any domain—whether music, athletics, or medicine. Didactics was wholly insufficient to describe what happened in simulation, which was a form of experiential learning, widely associated with work by educational theorist David Kolb (1984). Gallo liked the metaphor of a child learning to ride a bicycle: "Your parents didn't bring you into the living room and give you a PowerPoint presentation and a lecture." The educational methodology used throughout health care, which usually involved lectures and slideshow demonstrations, would not assign value to simulation much less lay down a path to its effective application.

Central to simulation, as Gallo and others in the field discovered, was the concept of *deliberate practice* (Ericsson, 1993). Developed during the 1990s by K. Anders Ericsson, a Swedish-born psychologist at the University of Florida, it provided a critique of the received wisdom around expert performance. Then the generally accepted view was that people reach a "stable asymptotic level" in learning beyond which they do not improve; the limits of mastery are genetically determined; and length of experience in a given field can account for level of expertise.

Ericsson developed an alternative view that was rooted in an empirical examination, first carried out with violinists and later extended to other domains, of how appropriate practice positively impacts performance. "Deliberate practice" was not the simple idea that "practice makes perfect" but, rather, the concept that educational activities can be designed to improve specific areas of performance. Violinists in Berlin, Ericsson and his colleagues discovered, "concentrated on improving specific aspects of the music performance as directed by their music teachers" (Ericsson, 2004, p. S73). He replicated his research with other musicians, notably pianists.

When he first discussed the concept of deliberate practice in relation to medicine in 2004, Ericsson in effect helped establish the mature framework for simulation. Setting out the goals of a scenario would mean watching for specific behaviors that indicated knowledge gaps or lack of expertise in specific areas that needed improvement. He pointed to the importance of immediate feedback and, discussing surgery, Ericsson recommended video recording "as is a common practice for enhancing the performance of athletes in soccer, football, and basketball" (Ericsson, 2004, p. S78). He noted that practice for rare events also represented acquisition of expertise. Debriefing, which would soon be developed more fully in terms of methods and aims (see Chapter 3), was in line with the same pedagogical philosophy.

ACQUIRING STAKEHOLDERS

Recognizing the underlying educational philosophy that simulation put into practice proved worthwhile in bringing PSI to the attention of early stakeholders. Not surprisingly, emergency medicine and family medicine, both specialties that tended to emphasize teamwork, turned out as early adopters; so, too, were departments of obstetrics/gynecology, a specialty in which patient satisfaction demanded nothing less than perfection. Neonatology and pediatrics would follow with a variety of specialized programs; so would behavioral health. Interprofessional teams would predominate in modeling programs, but there was also room for specialized group programs such as, in graduate medicine, cardiology fellows.

One early visitor to the institute was Alan Hartman, chairman of the Department of Cardiovascular and Thoracic Surgery at North Shore University Hospital. In terms of background and training, Hartman had no experience with simulation, and his zero exposure was the case with almost all physicians and surgeons trained in the 20th century. He had attended medical school from 1975 to 1979; his surgical internship and residency lasted until 1986. "The dictum of how you learned things then was 'See one, do one, teach one.' We had no simulation." When he toured PSI, Hartman was quick to recognize not only the possibilities for heart surgery and other cardiac interventions, but also its advantages in terms of de-emphasizing the hierarchy gradient and empowering all clinicians on a team. He could foresee that other clinical disciplines and specialties would eventually realize its multiple advantages. "In my education, my experience, we had none of this."

Hartman soon developed an initiative at both North Shore University Hospital and at Long Island Jewish Medical Center. Both cardiothoracic intensive care units (CT-ICUs) had good safety records but he was concerned about optimum response to rare cardiac emergencies. "We could have been a little bit better oiled machine." He understood how, ironically, excellent outcomes meant fewer opportunities to contend with emergencies, and he wanted to improve the communications skills and comfort level of his staff in dealing with them. In collaboration with PSI, he started to rotate teams of surgeons, intensivists, physician assistants, and critical care nurses through the simulation laboratory on a routine basis.

Collaboration between Hartman and the PSI staff intensified with the planned inauguration of a new tertiary CT-ICU at the health system's Southside Hospital (see Chapter 4). In fall 2010 they launched an intensive educational program designed to improve communication and teamwork among all staff on the surgical and post operative teams—physicians, physician assistants, nurses, nurse practitioners, and respiratory therapists. The program, formally known as the Cardiothoracic Service Focus Group, included both complex simulation scenarios at PSI and on-site drills. Five months after submission of the final Certificate of Need, working on an accelerated timetable, the new unit opened in February 2011—on schedule and without incident. Hartman credited simulation with efficiencies in team building and performance, noting that a couple of years later, a nearby competing institution, with a similar plan and timetable for a CT-ICU, had still not succeeded in opening.

PSI accumulated stakeholders, like Hartman's cardiothoracic units, over the course of several years beginning in 2007, and it established programs for units located throughout the 14 hospitals that now comprised the NS-LIJ Health System. The system itself, during the first decade of the century, assumed its present shape and, on an organizational basis, consolidated its identity. With more than 2,600 full-time physicians, residents, and fellows, and 6,000 community physicians, it became the nation's third-largest nonprofit, secular health system, as measured by beds; it was the fourteenth largest, based on patient revenue; and its research arm was the Feinstein Institute. Today it is the largest health system in New York State.

In response to demand from within the various NS-LIJ hospitals, PSI programs and staff expanded rapidly; by 2009 the institute had moved again and was physically housed with CLI. Soon it contemplated a further expansion effort that would involve creating an entirely new simulation space, together with a clinical skills center for teaching and assessment with standardized patients. The magnitude of that next incarnation owed in part to the fact that, beginning in 2011, PSI would take on another role—and an integral one—when institutional collaboration with Hofstra University established, from the ground up, a new 4-year medical school.

FURTHER EXPANSION AND OPENING TO MEDICAL EDUCATION

This is not the place to discuss in any detail the founding of the Hofstra-North Shore-LIJ School of Medicine, but several aspects deserve attention in passing— first, because plans for the school impacted PSI in terms of the shape of the fourth expansion in 5 years, and, in addition, because its complementary educational philosophy could help impart synergy to the health system as a whole.

Creating the medical school represented a response to a national call for more physicians in the United States; it was to be the first new one to open in New York State in 40 years. The proposed school's collaborative business structure, if not unique, was uncommon. Universities are the sole proprietors of the great majority of the country's medical schools and, through contractual arrangement with hospitals, they create internship and residency structures. By contrast, the Hofstra-North Shore-LIJ School of Medicine would be owned by its own health system, which offered the nearly unique opportunity to create a curriculum that made both creative use of the clinical services and drew upon faculty in clinical positions within it.

The school's corporate structure reflected the health system/university collaboration: Lawrence G. Smith, to become dean of the school, was also executive vice president and physician-in-chief of NS-LIJ; David Battinelli, to become dean for medical education, also served as the system's chief medical officer. To help develop the curriculum and its underlying conceptual foundation, between 2008 and 2010 they visited more than a dozen universities and medical schools in the United States and in Europe.

The result—the school opened its 4-year program in 2011—was an innovative curricular design, drawing upon models for contemporary business and law schools that inject real-world experience into the classroom from the first days of matriculation. The Hofstra-North Shore-LIJ School of Medicine dispensed with the traditional "two-by-two" model (basic science for 2 years, then 2 years of clinical medicine), which had become standard in medical schools during the 1970s and, although often criticized, has since been subject to only piecemeal reform. In place of this older structure, Smith and Battinelli developed a curriculum that propelled students into clinical work from the start. At the same time they entirely dispensed with classroom lectures, multiple choice exams, and intra-student competition. They abjured letter grades in favor of a pass-fail system that provided students with consistent evaluation and longitudinal tracking of achievement. This radical revision of the curriculum, which at the same time was consonant with much current academic thinking concerning medical education (Cooke, Irby, O'Brien, Carnegie Foundation for the Advancement of Teaching, & Ebrary Inc., 2010; Miller, Moore, Stead, & Balser, 2010; O'Connell & Pascoe, 2004), also aligned in multiple ways with the underlying principles of experiential learning that shaped PSI (Hirschman Miller & Battinelli, 2010).

So PSI, prior to the school's inaugural class in 2011, underwent a further expansion. Gallo and colleagues supervised construction. Although sheer size is no guarantee of quality—one competent simulation center noted in the literature measured approximately the size of a storeroom closet—they were provided with an additional 30,000 square feet, for a total of 45,000, making it one of the largest (Olympio, 2009). It included hospital rooms, surgical suites, control booths, and debriefing rooms arranged in modular fashion, equipped for audio and video recording and immediate playback; there was also an operating room with multiple cameras. In line with contemporary logistics, there were classrooms, small group rooms, a library, and "breakout spaces" (Horley, 2008), and an innovation café. Located within PSI was the new Clinical Skills Center for simulation with standardized patients. Overall, the larger institute could now respond to both the requirements of the new medical school and growing demand from the health system. Underscoring its strategic importance, Barbara DeVoe continued as director but was also promoted to Vice President for Interprofessional Learning and Education. Designed for efficiency and flexibility, the center opened in 2010.

Playing salient roles in both learning and assessment, PSI became for the students an integral part of the medical school, with the Center for Learning and Innovation designated as the school's West Campus. Simulation activities included extensive learning of clinical skills with standardized patients and high-fidelity simulation activities, but it also provided structures for curricular learning and for regular assessment. Students worked in teams and the institute also served as the place where through simulation they learned substantial aspects of basic science, including pathophysiology and pharmacology. Concomitant exposure to clinical scenarios in simulated environments represented an effort to inculcate habits of reflective practice early in a student's introduction to the culture of health care (Boutin-Foster, Foster, & Konopasek, 2008; Schön, 1983).

CULTURE OF SAFETY

The concept of a "culture of safety" was present but not fully defined in *To Err Is Human,* a document no less consistently cited in the literature today than was Abraham Flexner's 1910 report on medical education over much of the 20th century (Cooke, Irby, Sullivan, & Ludmerer, 2006). The authors explicitly referenced "culture" though they did not discuss what it meant in depth, probably owing to their broad charge to describe, for a wide audience, the stark state of affairs in health care. But the implications that flowed from recommendations in *To Err Is Human* were concrete and clearly stated (Kohn et al., 2000). Health organizations were in principle to "create a learning environment" to use simulation "whenever possible" and to "develop a working culture in which communication flows freely regardless of authority gradient" (p. 178). Feedback mechanisms had to be implemented and the success of CRM techniques in surgery and emergency medicine meant that "they should be more widely applied" (p. 179).

Building a health system that was imbued with those principles, however, and actually creating a genuine culture of safety was something else. It called for concrete steps and tasks that ranged across all clinical domains. Although much discussed from various angles in the contemporary literature, that task has proved long in the making (Chassin, 2013). Together with the other groups, organizations, and institutes that have come together over the first decade of the 21st century to advance patient safety through simulation, PSI forms part of a larger movement (Bradley, 2006). On a macro scale, this effort to create a culture of safety, with specific aims and standards, is developing rapidly. The Society for Simulation in Healthcare (SSH)—one of several such organizations—was established in 2004 with fewer than 200 members; by 2012 there were more than 3,000 (Gaba, 2013).

Viewed from its conceptual foundation and in terms of its design with respect to the larger organization that became the NS-LIJ Health System, PSI also represented an early 21st-century example of *systems integration* (Dunn, Deutsch, Maxworthy, Gallo, & Dong, 2013). A concept that refers to focused engineering approaches that globally impact the way an organization functions, systems integration readily applies to contemporary health care, owing to the multiple interconnected components of institutional providers; indeed, SSH includes it as an accreditation standard for organizations.

From its inception, PSI was conceived as a strategic means to use education to enhance both quality of care and patient safety throughout a large and expanding health care system. As a distinctive model, it is too soon to quantify its advantages or, indeed, judge its ultimate success, but its rapid establishment and growth can be understood as closely linked to engaging the goals of learning and the aspirations of CLI, the corporate university, and its parent organization. Historically, those goals and objectives should be understood as themselves the contingent outcome of rational decisions to suffuse the multihospital system and its human resources with concrete, culture-driven commitments to patient safety and to the transformative role of adult education and experiential learning.

NOTE

In addition to citations referenced below, this chapter is based on interviews the author conducted with David Battinelli, MD (11/26/2012; 10/4/2013); Barbara DeVoe, RN, DNP, FNP-BC, (12/13/2012; 9/11/2013); Kathleen Gallo, PhD, MBA, RN, FAAN (10/10/2012; 12/2/2012; 9/4/2013); Alan Hartman, MD (3/7/2013); and Lawrence G. Smith, MD, MACP (10/16/2012).

REFERENCES

Assen, D. (2010). *Corporate Universities: Making a strategic contribution by enhancing absorptive capacity.* Paper presented at the proceedings of the International HRD conference, Pecs, Hungary.

Blouin, A. S., & McDonagh, K. J. (2011). Framework for patient safety, part 1: Culture as an imperative. *Journal of Nursing Administration, 41*(10), 397–400. doi:10.1097/NNA.0b013e31822edb4d

Boutin-Foster, C., Foster, J. C., & Konopasek, L. (2008). Viewpoint: Physician, know thyself: The professional culture of medicine as a framework for teaching cultural competence. *Academic Medicine, 83*(1), 106–111. doi:10.1097/ACM.0b013e31815c6753

Bower, J., & Christensen, C. (1995). Disruptive technologies: Catching the wave. *Harvard Business Review, 73*(1), 43–53. doi:citeulike-article-id:4498915

Bradley, P. (2006). The history of simulation in medical education and possible future directions. *Medical Education, 40*(3), 254–262. doi:10.1111/j.1365-2929.2006.02394.x

Chassin, M. R. (2013). Improving the quality of health care: What's taking so long? *Health Affairs (Millwood), 32*(10), 1761–1765. doi:10.1377/hlthaff.2013.0809

Cooke, M., Irby, D. M., O'Brien, B. C., Carnegie Foundation for the Advancement of Teaching, & Ebrary Inc. (2010). *Educating physicians: A call for reform of medical school and residency. Preparation for the professions series.* Retrieved from http://site.ebrary.com/lib/berkeley/Doc?id=10388359

Cooke, M., Irby, D. M., Sullivan, W., & Ludmerer, K. M. (2006). American medical education 100 years after the Flexner report. *The New England Journal of Medicine, 355*(13), 1339–1344. doi:10.1056/NEJMra055445

Cooper, J. B., & Taqueti, V. R. (2004). A brief history of the development of mannequin simulators for clinical education and training. *Quality & Safety in Health Care, 13*(Suppl. 1), i11–i18. doi:10.1136/qhc.13.suppl_1.i11

Dowling, M. (2001). *The North Shore-LIJ Leadership Institute.* Unpublished White Paper.

Dunn, W., Deutsch, E. S., Maxworthy, J., Gallo, K., & Dong, Y. (2013). Systems integration. In A. I. Levine (Ed.), *Comprehensive textbook of healthcare simulation.* New York, NY: Springer.

Ericsson, K. A. (1993). The role of deliberate practice in the acquisition of expert performance. *Psychological Review, 100*(3), 363–406.

Ericsson, K. A. (2004). Deliberate practice and the acquisition and maintenance of expert performance in medicine and related domains. *Academic Medicine, 79*(Suppl. 10), S70–S81.

Friedman, M. I., Cooper, A. H., Click, E., & Fitzpatrick, J. J. (2011). Specialized new graduate RN critical care orientation: Retention and financial impact. *Nursing Economics, 29*(1), 7–14.

Friedman, M. I., Delaney, M. M., Schmidt, K., Quinn, C., & Macyk, I. (2013). Specialized new graduate RN pediatric orientation: A strategy for nursing retention and its financial impact. *Nursing Economics, 31*(4), 162–170; quiz 171.

Gaba, D. (2013). Foreward. In A. I. Levine, S. DeMaria Jr., A. D. Schwartz, A. J. Sim (Eds.), *The comprehensive textbook of healthcare simulation* (pp. vii). New York, NY: Springer

Gaba, D. M. (2004). The future vision of simulation in health care. *Quality & Safety in Health Care, 13*(Suppl. 1), i2–i10. doi:10.1136/qhc.13.suppl_1.i2

Gaba, D. M., Howard, S. K., Fish, K. J., Smith, B. E., & Sowb, Y. A. (2001). Simulation-based training in anesthesia crisis resource management (ACRM): A decade of experience. *Simulation & Gaming, 32*(2), 175–193.

Gardner, R., & Raemer, D. B. (2008). Simulation in obstetrics and gynecology. *Obstetrics and Gynecology Clinics of North America, 35*(1), 97–127, ix. doi:10.1016/j.ogc.2007.12.008

GE Crotonville. (n.d.). Retrieved from http://www.ge.com/careers/culture/university-students

Gebauer, J., Lowman, D., & Gordon, J. (2008). *Closing the engagement gap: How great companies unlock employee potential for superior results.* New York, NY: Portfolio.

Helmreich, R. L. (2000). On error management: Lessons from aviation. *BMJ, 320*(7237), 781–785.

Hirschman Miller, E., & Battinelli, D. (2010). Association of American Medical Colleges predicts decreased number of US-trained physicians: Profiling the response of Hofstra University School of Medicine in partnership with North Shore-Long Island Jewish Health System. *Postgraduate Medicine, 122*(4), 232–233. doi:10.3810/pgm.2010.07.2194

Horley, R. (2008). Simulation and skill centre design. In R. Riley (Ed.), *Manual of simulation in healthcare* (pp. 3–10). New York, NY: Oxford University Press.

Institute of Medicine. (2003). *Health professions education: A bridge to quality.* Washington, DC: Author.

Issenberg, S. B., McGaghie, W. C., Petrusa, E. R., Lee Gordon, D., & Scalese, R. J. (2005). Features and uses of high-fidelity medical simulations that lead to effective learning: A BEME systematic review. *Medical Teacher, 27*(1), 10–28. doi:10.1080/01421590500046924

Jeffries, P. R. (2009). Dreams for the future for clinical simulation. *Nursing Education Perspectives, 30*(2), 71.

Kerner, R. (2010). *Creating an interdisciplinary simulation center. High-fidelity patient simulation in nursing education* (p. xxii). Sudbury, MA: Jones and Bartlett.

Kohn, L. T., Corrigan, J., & Donaldson, M. S. (2000). *To err is human: Building a safer health system.* Washington, DC: National Academy Press.

Kolb, D. A. (1984). *Experiential learning: Experience as the source of learning and development.* Englewood Cliffs, NJ: Prentice-Hall.

Lampotang, S. (2008). Medium and high integration mannequin patient simulators. In R. H. Riley (Ed.), *Manual of simulation in healthcare* (pp. 51–64). Oxford, England: Oxford University Press.

Leape, L. L., & Berwick, D. M. (2005). Five years after to err is human: What have we learned? *JAMA: The Journal of the American Medical Association, 293*(19), 2384–2390. doi:10.1001/jama.293.19.2384

Miller, B. M., Moore, D. E., Jr., Stead, W. W., & Balser, J. R. (2010). Beyond Flexner: A new model for continuous learning in the health professions. *Academic Medicine, 85*(2), 266–272. doi:10.1097/ACM.0b013e3181c859fb

Naik, V. N., & Brien, S. E. (2013). Review article: Simulation: A means to address and improve patient safety. *Canadian Journal of Anaesthesia, 60*(2), 192–200. doi:10.1007/s12630-012-9860-z

O'Connell, M. T., & Pascoe, J. M. (2004). Undergraduate medical education for the 21st century: Leadership and teamwork. *Family Medicine, 36*(Suppl.), S51–S56.

Olympio, M. A. (2009). Space considerations in health care simulation. In G.E. Loyd, C. L. Lake, & R. B. Greenberg (Eds.), *Practical health care simulations.* Philadelphia, PA: Elsevier.

Peter M. (n.d.). *Winter institute for simulation education and research.* Retrieved from http://www.wiser.pitt.edu/sites/wiser/aboutus/history.asp

Rosen, K. R. (2008). The history of medical simulation. *Journal of Critical Care, 23*(2), 157–166. doi:10.1016/j.jcrc.2007.12.004

Schön, D. A. (1983). *The reflective practitioner: How professionals think in action.* New York, NY: Basic Books.

Society for Simulation in Healthcare. (2013). Interprofessional Education and Healthcare Simulation Symposium.

Stelfox, H. T., Palmisani, S., Scurlock, C., Orav, E. J., & Bates, D. W. (2006). The "To err is human" report and the patient safety literature. *Quality & Safety in Health Care, 15*(3), 174–178. doi:10.1136/qshc.2006.017947

Stevens, R. (1989). *In sickness and in wealth: American hospitals in the twentieth century.* New York, NY: Basic Books.

Wallace, P. (1997). Following the threads of an innovation: The history of standardized patients in medical education. *Caduceus, 13*(2), 5–28.

Zink, B. J. (2006). *Anyone, anything, anytime: a history of emergency medicine* (1st ed.). Philadelphia, PA: Mosby Elsevier.

Barbara DeVoe
Robert L. Kerner Jr.

2: Practical and Tactical Aspects of Debriefing

Understood as the "heart and soul" of medical simulation, successful debriefing requires that facilitators acquire a skillset that is widely acknowledged to be elusive and difficult to master. This chapter examines the development of debriefing from a historical perspective and provides practical guidance for clinical educators. Based on extensive experience, it draws on some of the underlying medico-sociological and psychological models to suggest concrete methods by which facilitators can develop and consistently apply a basic viewpoint that favors inquisitiveness and curiosity while relying on evidence-based standards of care in clinical medicine and scientific data to help participants and teams close the great variety of gaps in knowledge, performance, skills, and attitude revealed during simulation.

A SHORT HISTORY OF FACILITATED DEBRIEFING

The process that today we call debriefing was originally developed in the military and referred to the method by which former hostages and prisoners of war could provide useful information and insight by detailing their experiences, with a view to improving both operations and strategy (Dismukes & McDonnell, 1997; Fanning & Gaba, 2007). There subsequently developed the therapeutic concept of "critical incident stress debriefing" (CISD) led by a "facilitator," which eventually also found uses in disaster management as a means to avoid or mitigate, at least in principle, posttraumatic psychopathology (Mitchell, 1983). Psychologists also adopted the concept to help participants in their experiments, which often involved deception, escape harm by revealing "what really happened" (Fanning & Gaba, 2007; Lederman, 1992). Uses for debriefing in psychology have continued to advance over several decades, with various applications in response to emergency and traumatic situations (Choe, 2005).

As applied to simulation in medicine, however, the field of experiential learning provides the most germane context to consider debriefing. Beginning in the early 1980s, communications experts recognized the potential and broad applicability of simulation to education—most especially for adults. Linda Lederman undertook to sort out its various components and defined it as "a process by which people who have had an experience are led through a purposive discussion of that experience" (Lederman, 1992, p. 146). She understood the relevance of debriefing in helping to fulfill cognitive, affective, and behavioral objectives, and she explicitly connected it to the sorts of educational reform advocated early in the 20th century by John Dewey. Debriefing, asserted Lederman, "is an integral part of any learning experience that is designed to be experience based" (Lederman, 1992, p. 158).

Like other components of simulation, debriefing actually entered medicine and medical education via adaptation of safety programs created first by group leaders in the field of military aviation and the airline industry. Post-crash investigations of airplane disasters in the 1970s revealed that neither mechanical malfunction nor the competency of individual members of the flight crew were responsible (Dismukes, Gaba, & Howard, 2006). Rather, the root cause was most frequently impaired or dysfunctional communication, including flight crew failures to share information. Subsequent development and application of "crew resource management" (CRM) to flight simulation activities included post-hoc "debriefings" specifically designed to improve the technical skills and interaction among crew members. From the beginning, CRM tenets stressed the centrality of the debrief. The instructor was "expected to encourage the crewmembers to analyze their . . . performance on their own, rather than lecturing to them about what they did right and wrong" (Dismukes & McDonnell, 1997, p. 1). It was a "crew-centered approach" that emphasized "self-discovery and self-critique" (Dismukes & McDonnell 1997, p. 1).

In the late 1980s, David Gaba and colleagues at Stanford University emerged as the principal architects of renewed interest in high-fidelity, manikin-based medical simulation (Bradley, 2006; Howard, Gaba, Fish, Yang, & Sarnquist, 1992; Rosen, 2008). An anesthesiologist with a degree in bioengineering, Gaba adopted the principles of CRM for a team training approach with simulation scenarios. Courses in anesthesia crisis resource management (ACRM) from the start recognized that the debrief could be described as "the most important component" of the experience, which closely followed the lead set out by the aviation model:

> With guidance from the instructor, [members of the team] link their observations to behaviors and events from the real world. Instructors strive for an atmosphere of constructive critique and feedback provided in a supportive, nonjudgmental manner. They aim for

maximum participant involvement, open-ended questioning, and active learning. Ideally, the instructor should merely facilitate the process of the group debriefing itself. (Gaba, Fish, Smith, & Sowb, 2001, p. 182)

Although CRM principles initially set out to create a new learning environment in anesthesiology, the scope of high-fidelity simulation dramatically expanded over the course of a decade, and by the turn of the century efforts were under way for use with health care providers in intensive care units, emergency and trauma departments, cardiac response teams, perinatal care, and radiology (Gaba, 2001). In anesthesiology, simulation and consequent interest in debriefing have continued to grow and become part of an international effort to improve patient safety (Flin, Patey, Glavin, & Maran, 2010).

With respect to debriefing, Gaba and his colleagues followed in the footsteps of Lederman in seeking to square the basic concepts of CRM with contemporary educational theory. They pointed to David Kolb's description of the "experiential learning cycle" and, as a helpful corrective, Graham Gibbs's "reflective learning cycle"; the latter explicitly specifically embraced debriefing (Gibbs, 1988; Kolb, 1984). The various models, Gaba suggested, "probably all evolve out of the natural order of human processing to experience an event, to reflect on it, to discuss it with others, and learn and modify behaviors based on the experience" (Fanning & Gaba, 2007, p. 117). The debrief, that is, was understood to be a conversation, facilitated but not directed as a top-down exercise. It was not only a cognitive enterprise, but also involved "learning by doing," as Gibbs noted, and it paid attention to emotional and interactive features of education with a view to long-lasting knowledge acquisition.

The transfer of skills and knowledge about debriefings to the facilitators who actually conduct them presented a challenge from the beginning—and continues to do so today (Flanagan, 2008). For most, with the exception of professionals at dedicated simulation centers, it is a part-time or incidental occupation. Facilitators are generally supervising nurses, physicians, and physician assistants. Although principles of reflective learning can be explained to them through didactic work and practice sessions, how should facilitators understand their role? How, in concrete terms, should they carry it out? In terms of medical education, most have been trained in silos rather than interprofessional contexts, and traditional instruction, like that in other skill-based professions, has typically involved a top-down approach to learning and assessment of performance. Debriefing, however, has always been understood to be learner-centric and learner-based (Lederman, 1992). Flanagan describes the tendency for facilitators and learners to conduct themselves as though in a classroom in which the teacher-as-debriefer "controls the agenda and the learners sit passively, too timid to speak." It is a "temptation," he notes, that "must be resisted" (Flanagan, 2008, p. 157).

A variety of tools are available to help orient and instruct facilitators (Hart, McNeil, Griswold-Theodorson, Bhatia, & Joing, 2012; Overstreet, 2010; Owen & Follows, 2006; Salas et al., 2008). We might note, just as an example, the useful basic mnemonic known as DEBRIEF, associated with the U.S. Army's After Action Review:

D = Define the rules of the debriefing session
E = Explain the learning objectives
B = Benchmark performance: explain what the standard is
R = Review what was supposed to happen in the scenario
I = Identify what actually happened
E = Examine why things happened the way they did; what were the performance gaps
F = Formalize learning points so participants leave with a clear understanding of what to do next time

The explicit requirements of "E" and ""B" to set out learning objectives and explain performance benchmarks, we have found, help to ensure that key elements to orient participants are in place prior to the simulation.

Perhaps the most developed and cogent effort to provide a reasonable schemata for debriefing, both faithful to experiential learning theory and rooted in experience, emerged from the Center for Medical Simulation at Harvard Medical School in 2006, with publication by Jenny Rudolph and colleagues in the paper entitled, "There's No Such Thing as 'Nonjudgmental" Debriefing: A Theory and Method for Debriefing with Good Judgment" (Rudolph, Simon, Dufresne, & Raemer, 2006). Based upon the concept of "reflective practice" as first developed by Donald Schön in the 1970s, which found some success in business education and was familiar to many in the health care professions, the Harvard group provided both a theoretical model and, at least in principle, a practical method (Schön, 1983). Rooted in cognitive science, "debriefing with good judgment" employs the notion that internal mental "frames," which hypothetically consist of trainees' knowledge, assumptions, and feelings, drive the way that they act and interact during simulation. Facilitators (or instructors) could conduct debriefings in ways that would not involve punitive and damaging judgments of performance while at the same time avoiding equally ineffective sugar-coated critiques with the simple hope that participants will self-correct and learn by doing. By adopting a basic stance of "genuine curiosity," the facilitator's role is to discern these frames and employ a conversational technique, known as "advocacy and inquiry" that pairs an assertion or observation (which implies a hypothesis) to be in effect tested with a conversational question. The aim is to promote a self-reflective evaluative judgment that fosters learning and change while remaining within a context of respect and collaboration. Debriefing With Good Judgment represents the most prominent of several efforts to resolve a basic dilemma facing the simulation community as it intersects with the patient safety movement to substantively address the "iceberg of errors" in medicine. But, as was noted at the time, "Translating the theoretical ideas in the paper of Rudolph, et al., into the practical conduct of debriefings may not be easy, even for instructors who are already familiar with facilitated debriefing." (Dismukes et al., 2006, p. 24)

Accordingly, in the following we formulate some broad strategies and concrete tactics for facilitators. As suggestions, they draw to some extent on medico–sociological and psychological concepts, but for the most part they represent a distillation of experience, the practical yield from thousands of simulation sessions—rising to more than 50,000 learner hours in 2013—both with health care personnel from a large nonprofit hospital and with students from an undergraduate medical education program.

Practical and Tactical Aspects

Facilitators, who are often teachers in other venues, must above all change and recast their mental models of what it means to be an instructor in a debriefing. Models of conventional didactics do not apply. A debriefing is not the place to teach the fundamental principles of oxygenation, for example; but it is the place to be inquisitive about what learners know about those principles and how they might apply in a particular scenario, and to be sure that they leave with the learning objectives met and knowledge assimilated. The aim is not to grill learners or to question their judgment and behaviors; it is rather to inquire about what they do, to validate their knowledge and understanding, and, if need be, to point them in the right direction.

Preparations for debriefings begin ahead of simulation. Facilitators may need to introduce themselves, orient participants to the locale or surroundings, and provide any logistical details that will help make participants comfortable. The tone throughout should be conversational. Facilitators should explain in general terms the rationale for the simulation together with an opening statement that outlines the common platform—that is, what is expected of participants. In a high-fidelity context, for example:

Facilitator: In our simulation today I want you to do everything that you would ordinarily do for a patient in the hospital. Whatever you would do or say to a patient, you should do or say to the manikin.

Debriefs examine and reflect on what transpires in simulation sessions across three major categories or domains. The first, *teamwork and communication,* includes both behavior among team members and interactions with the patient, whether a manikin or a standardized patient. *Clinical treatment* is the second broad domain, for which facilitators must silently pose to themselves the question: Are team members individually and collectively doing the right thing and for the right reasons? Finally, debriefs will include assessment of *general situational awareness.* Do team members know what is happening in their immediate environment, and are they anticipating what might happen as a consequence of their actions?

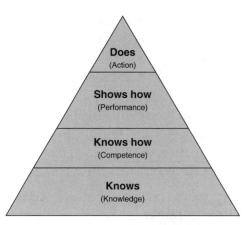

FIGURE 2.1 Miller's assessment pyramid. Miller (1990). Used by permission.

In terms of assessing competency, facilitators might consider that the sort of assessment in the advocacy/inquiry model, described above, corresponds in basic outline to the "shows how" layer of Miller's Pyramid/Prism (Figure 2.1; Miller, 1990). Briefly put, the learners' ability to integrate knowledge is what facilitators look for in every debriefing. Do participants understand the basic science? Do they know what to do with it? Do they know how to act and when to act? Do their physical dexterity and actions align with their knowledge? Last, but not least, can participants communicate with team members to ensure that interventions are safe and effective?

The Basic Shift: From Observation to Inquiry As the simulation session ends and participants gather to debrief, the facilitator's basic stance undergoes a self-conscious cognitive shift from critical observation to curiosity and genuine inquisitiveness. To borrow from the language of phenomenology, sometimes used with reference to qualitative research (Creswell, 2007), the facilitator "brackets" or puts aside assumptions and judgments. Drawing no conclusions at the outset enables the facilitator to formulate a small set of observations and questions that derive first of all from the preexisting learning objectives and, second, from the session as it actually transpired. The verbal and physical behaviors that the facilitator observes are treated as raw data to be investigated against the backdrop of a scenario constructed with several specific learning objectives. Assumptions concerning mistakes, whether omissions or committed errors, are put on hold in favor of observation and associated queries. An example in simplest form:

Facilitator: I noticed you put the [AED] pads on upside down. So what made you do that?

In terms of the advocacy/inquiry model, the observation represents advocacy—there is a right way and wrong way to apply the pads—while the question expresses an inquiry that avoids a harsh and potentially counterproductive judgment. Underlying both statements is the stance of genuine curiosity that aims to discover what the participants were thinking and doing during the simulation, and why. Often enough, assumptions that facilitators make concerning apparent mistakes on the part of individuals or teams during simulations are wrong. Curiosity helps reveal the hidden mental "frames" that shape thought and action (Rudolph, Simon, Raemer, & Eppich, 2008). For a facilitator, naiveté is a virtue.

Recourse to Science and Accepted Best Practice One benefit of reserving judgment concerning correspondence errors observed during simulation is that facilitators can bring scientific and clinical issues to the foreground, unburdened by hierarchical authority. In several specific ways, they can help the debriefing conversation explore, discover, and resolve gaps or lacunae in individual and team knowledge, performance, skills, and attitudes.

Knowledge gaps occur when behavior during simulation represents mental frames that depart from what is currently known, research-based, and forms part of the accepted standard of care. Such gaps may owe to aspects of care that simply have not been learned or were wrongly learned or forgotten. People may have acted in accordance with an institutional norm that is outdated or surpassed by new knowledge, or by technology that embodies new knowledge. Still others may be due to anachronistic beliefs or practices associated with long-standing controversial issues.

Oxygen therapy and adequate ventilation, for example, are central to emergency care today, based on recognition of clinical features. At the same time, whether oxygen may cause carbon dioxide retention in emergency patients with chronic obstructive pulmonary disease (COPD) is a long-debated issue and may be misinterpreted in ways that cause undue delay or reluctance to employ it (Murphy, Driscoll, & O'Driscoll, 2001). With open-ended questions and a minimum of guidance, facilitators can probe such issues during debriefs and, if necessary, ensure that in the end participants come away with messages that align with the standard of care:

Facilitator: Just so we're all on the same page, the current standard of care is: give oxygen; put the patient on a ventilator if need be.

Performance gaps refer to behavior, including verbal behavior, that potentially or actually adversely affect teamwork and patient care. In a surgical safety simulation, for example, protocol for a laterality check might require the surgeon to mark the site of the forthcoming procedure, to be confirmed by the anesthesiologist. Suppose instead, during simulation, the anesthesiologist enters the operating suite and asks the nursing personnel: "What knee are we operating on?" He then goes on to mark the knee itself together with the site on the hip where he would inject the anesthesia.

Facilitator: I saw you marked the knee. Tell us why you did that.
Anesthesiologist: I see everyone else in my department marking the knee.
Facilitator: Did you consider that a nurse might assume that the surgeon had marked the knee?
Anesthesiologist: I never thought of that.

Skills and attitude gaps often occur when behavior in a simulation runs counter to accepted standard of care and owes to personal preference, idiosyncrasy, or misaligned commitment. These represent a type of knowledge gap that can lead to hostile interchanges and must be carefully managed.

To cite an example from cardiac resuscitation, use of a backboard is generally recommended and recent studies using high-fidelity simulation show that, especially on mattress surfaces, it increases the effectiveness of chest compression and provides support for the spine. When during simulation a nurse suggested its use to the physician assistant who had taken charge of the team, the following exchange occurred during simulation:

Physician Assistant: It's a waste of time.
Nurse: [Repeated, while holding the backboard] We should use the backboard.
Physician Assistant: Get out of here. It's an utter waste of time.

It is worth noting that strong emotions generally, including anger, indicate a useful and desirable commitment to the simulation scenario; in general, facilitators should recognize that their mental models of what good learners look like do not always align with real-world experience. At the same time, hostility owing to a skills and attitude gap can spill over into the debrief and must be addressed:

Facilitator: I noticed that you rejected the idea of using a backboard.
Physician Assistant: I think it's an utter waste of time.
Facilitator: You said no to the backboard, so help me understand your decision.
Physician Assistant: People take forever to go find a backboard.
Facilitator: But in this case, the nurse was holding it in his hands.
Physician Assistant: It's stupid.

To resolve such conflicts in the debrief, which may be tinged with hostility or frustration and set one participant at odds with the team, facilitators may consider using the technique known as "normalization," by which they use the complaint itself to help probe for real-world patterns of behavior (Bartone, 1995; Foa, 2010).

Facilitator: I hear what you're saying. Is this a problem at the hospital?
Physician Assistant: All the time. None of the equipment is in the place where you'd normally find it. It's stupid.
Facilitator: How do you deal with it?
Physician Assistant: Maybe I'll send a nurse.
Facilitator: Did you consider doing that here?

Normalization—the term is often used in relation to posttraumatic stress disorder—avoids treating behaviors that require attention as symptoms denoting pathology. It also affords an opportunity to address such issues as the reluctance as a team member to speak up. To continue with the previous example:

Nurse Practitioner: I know that the backboard is standard. Why didn't I say anything to the PA [physician assistant]? I guess I didn't want to be wrong.

Facilitator: Why don't you want to be wrong? If you were wrong, what do you think would be the consequences?

Nurse Practitioner: The PA might yell at me.

Facilitator: Has he ever?

Nurse Practitioner: No. No one yells at me.

Facilitator: So that might not be realistic.

Nurse Practitioner: No. But I might feel bad.

Facilitator: Has that happened in some other part of your life? You were wrong and felt bad? How did you deal with it?

Nurse Practitioner: I guess you just move on. But I don't like feeling stupid in front of my peers.

Facilitator: Can you weigh what's more important? Your peers being critical of you or the outcome of the treatment you're providing the patient?

Helping participants resolve these and similar issues along the largely non-directive lines of adult learning favors the development of good judgment in interprofessional contexts.

Resolve Conflict by Identifying Fundamental Attribution Errors Debriefings can sometimes reveal simmering and submerged tensions among members of health care teams. Whether they owe to classic adversarial tensions as described in the literature (Blickensderfer, 1996; Kelly, 2006; Leever et al., 2010) or more simply to past behaviors that are misinterpreted or distorted, they can be addressed when revealed during debriefing. In a case of potential cardiac arrest in a coronary care unit, for example, consider a simulation that played out during which the team failed to telephone the cardiologist, who was observing the session. During the debrief, he expressed his anger and received a sharp response:

Cardiologist: Why the hell don't you call me? I was at home, not on the moon. It was eleven o'clock at night, but no matter. Why don't you nurses ever call me?

Nurse: You want to know why? When we called you late at night 2 years ago, you were rude to us. And no one wants to suffer your attitude on the telephone.

The mood of the debriefing room in such situations can be tense and facilitators will often find that silence is a valuable response. In this case, the interchange created an opportunity to identify dueling attribution errors.

Cardiologist: Do you know why I got upset? I'll explain it to you.

He proceeded to tell a story about a patient who was extremely sick. The nursing staff took time compiling extraneous information, and when they reached him by phone they conveyed it all before noting that the patient was virtually in cardiac arrest. What he wanted to hear was, "Cardiac arrest. You must come in." Instead, staff provided him with a lengthy presentation of nonessential information.

Two separate fundamental attribution errors may be identified. The surgeon, based on one or two phone calls that did not prioritize essential data, made the assumption that every nurse who called him at night would waste his time with information not germane to a crisis. For their part, the nurses made the assumption that the physician would respond to their calls with vituperation.

Employing Narrative and Story The cognitive theory that helps to frame the advocacy/inquiry model to be used in "debriefing with good judgment" makes use, as noted, of the concept of "internal frames" to describe a mental model which guides action. On a practical basis, facilitators are customarily counseled to begin a debriefing by testing or "viewing" these frames with simple open-ended questions concerning the simulation just completed:

Facilitator: So, what happened? How did it go?

It is worth recognizing that these questions represent invitations to provide an account or story, as a basic test of coherence in shared human communication. Although narrative in simulation generally takes place in a somewhat different register than that used in some nursing contexts (which emphasize empathy and shared meaning), it plays a central role in debriefing in several specific ways. Simulation scenarios themselves embody story elements aligned with learning objectives; it is generally the team's task to recognize salient aspects of the clinical situation and respond appropriately. "Narrative pedagogy" has an excellent fit with critical thinking as applied to debriefing (Rubenfield, 2005; Walsh, 2011).

Consider, for example, a high-fidelity simulation that involves a patient who presents with severe anaphylaxis. With symptoms that include angioedema, generalized urticaria, and history of allergy to bee sting, the diagnosis is fairly obvious. The facilitator, operating from a stance of genuine curiosity with the aim of helping to improve performance, asks for an explanation:

Facilitator: Help me understand what's going on. Can you explain to me the biochemical cascade? What's going on here?

The cascade, in its essential form a succession of biochemical events that can be readily described in a story format, may be included among the learning objectives in the preexisting scenario. The team may need to explain, for example, how antigen-preventing cells (APCs) fragment offending proteins in bee venom, which combine with human leukocyte antigens (HLAs) for presentation to leucocytes, and the resulting T-cell activation leads to cytokine release and the symptoms of anaphylaxis.

Facilitator: Now can you tell about what you did to take care of the patient and how your actions impacted the cascade? Assume I'm the patient and tell me why the treatment you gave (e.g., Benadryl and epinephrine) works for anaphylaxis. Tell me the story.

Requesting a narrative during a debriefing is a practical solution for a facilitator that encourages team communication and assimilation of knowledge while sidestepping any impulse to lecture. Narrative pedagogy in this sense becomes "a valuable tool that should be used in conjunction with a content and competency-driven curriculum" and aligns with simulation in opening up "new ways of learning and knowing and also helps to locate more traditional learning in the human complexity of the real world" (Walsh, 2011, p. 216).

A narrative approach also provides an opportunity to engage the more passive members of a team who tend to be quiet during debriefings. Facilitators are tasked with making sure that no one is left out of the debrief:

Facilitator [to the passive learner]: Anything more to add? Anything you'd do differently? What would you add to the story so far?

Use of Video Following up on the experience in aviation and CRM, the research by Gaba and colleagues that shaped the field of contemporary medical simulation employed video to record simulation sessions and to identify gaps in the training of anesthesiologists (Gaba et al., 2001). Audiovisual systems have subsequently become a common feature in simulation centers as an aid to debriefing. Today, they tend to be wholly computer-controlled, with digital capability to locate specific portions that can be instantly replayed. Although facilitators are apt not to resort to video segments in every debrief, and research regarding the value of video-assisted debriefing has yielded mixed results, the ability to examine snippets and short portions from a simulation in a mediated context is always a potentially valuable resource.

Like others in dedicated simulation centers, we have found video to be a useful adjunct when judiciously employed. In high-fidelity contexts it can provide teachable moments, illustrate obvious errors and omissions, and serve as confirmation of observed behavior. Video can also identify communication process gaps—failure to ask a crucial question owing to interference, for example—and it can eliminate arguments concerning who said what to whom. For evaluating performance during simulations that focus on communication with patients and family members, video-assisted debriefing can also provide immediate feedback to individuals and to teams. Video can not only show obvious errors in communication; it can also capture subtle shifts in voice patterns, body language, and other nonverbal cues.

Although video can be considered a tool to be used in debriefing, it should be no surprise that its value is limited. Debriefs are time-constrained and learner-centric, so facilitators need to respect the learning objectives of any particular scenario and remain aware of achieving balance in discussion. When standardized patients are used, their presence in the debrief can be helpful and in some measure obviate the importance of video recording. In addition, recording sound and visuals raises issues of confidentiality that should be addressed when orienting participants who need to feel confident their performances are not being evaluated outside the simulation context.

Research concerning the use of video in debriefing simulation has generated a variety of encouraging though sometimes mixed results. Studies in 2002 and 2003, for example, that investigate epidural analgesia and trauma resuscitation, respectively, were positive (Birnbach et al., 2002; Scherer, Chang, Meredith, & Battistella, 2003). However, a 2006 study by Savoldelli and colleagues that compared oral-assisted feedback, video-assisted oral feedback, and no feedback readily showed the value of debriefing but not the ancillary use of video (Savoldelli et al., 2006). More recently, a study of neonatal resuscitation showed the effect of video-assisted debriefing to be insignificant as compared with no video (Sawyer et al., 2012). In brief, no consensus exists as to the ultimate value of video in simulation or how it should be used for optimum results.

Instruments for Evaluating Debriefings Most facilitators are health care providers with supervisory responsibilities and may be considered stakeholders in the various units or departments whose personnel are participants in simulations. To learn the basic principles of debriefing, they undergo instruction and observation, optimally under the auspices of a simulation center, but practices vary widely.

Debriefing Assessment for Simulation in Healthcare (DASH) is the most comprehensive of several tools that aim to evaluate the quality of debriefs (Simon R., 2009). Created in conjunction with the Advocacy and Inquiry Model of Debriefing with Good Judgment, DASH is a generalized quality assurance and assessment tool developed by the Center for Medical Simulation (Boston). It may be used with a wide variety of disciplines and types of simulation. Six elements, each of them scored by a rater, examine concrete behaviors around experiential learning. Using a rating scale of 1 to 7 points, the various elements help evaluate the setting for the debrief, assess whether the overall context and structure are engaging, to what extent the discussion is conducive to reflective practice, and if it identifies and helps close performance gaps. In a study with participants that included nurses, physicians, and other health care professionals, Brett-Fleegler et al. have reported favorable results in terms of both reliability and validity (Brett-Fleegler et al., 2012). The tool itself includes useful descriptions and examples of the behaviors associated with each dimension ("Rater's Handbook—DASH" [2010]).

Implementation of DASH, however, is not always simple. In a complex health care environment with part-time facilitators who may only debrief a few hours each month, it can prove challenging. It may be labor intensive—particularly if raters work with a video-recorded debrief to provide feedback—and may require extra time from personnel.

Concluding Remarks

Although debriefing has long been an integral component of simulation, whether high-fidelity or with standardized patients, adapting it for use in medicine presented a number of distinctive challenges. The breadth and depth of the ever-expanding knowledge base and the burden of education in silos count for two; many more might be cited. But the past decade has seen development of a variety of useful tools and strategies—some discussed here—that ensure debriefing helps to bring about the substantial advances in patient safety that are at the heart of simulation (Salas, Wilson, Burke, & Priest, 2005). Research thus far consistently demonstrates the value of facilitated conversation to simulation, and future efforts are likely to fine tune its range of tactics and make further and measurable advances in efficacy (Gaba, 2004; Issenberg, McGaghie, Petrusa, Lee Gordon, & Scalese, 2005; McGaghie, Issenberg, Petrusa, & Scalese, 2010).

REFERENCES

Bartone, P. T., & Alder, A. B. (1995). *Event-oriented debriefing following military operations: What every leader should know*. Ft. Detrick, Frederick, MD: US Army Medical Research & Materiel Command.

Birnbach, D. J., Santos, A. C., Bourlier, R. A., Meadows, W. E., Datta, S., Stein, D. J., . . . Thys, D. M. (2002). The effectiveness of video technology as an adjunct to teach and evaluate epidural anesthesia performance skills. *Anesthesiology, 96*(1), 5–9.

Blickensderfer, L. (1996). Nurses and physicians: creating a collaborative environment. *Journal of Intravenous Nursing, 19*(3), 127–131.

Bradley, P. (2006). The history of simulation in medical education and possible future directions. *Medical Education, 40*(3), 254–262. doi:10.1111/j.1365-2929.2006.02394.x

Brett-Fleegler, M., Rudolph, J., Eppich, W., Monuteaux, M., Fleegler, E., Cheng, A., & Simon, R. (2012). Debriefing assessment for simulation in healthcare: Development and psychometric properties. *Simulation in Healthcare, 7*(5), 288–294. doi:10.1097/SIH.0b013e3182620228

Choe, I. (2005). The debate over psychological debriefing for PTSD. *New School Psychology Bulletin, 3*(2), 71–82.

Creswell, J. W. (2007). *Qualitative inquiry and research design*. Thousand Oaks CA: Sage.

Dismukes, J. K., & McDonnell, L. K. (1997). *Facilitating LOS debriefings: A training manual*. Moffett Field, CA: NASA's Ames Research Center.

Dismukes, R. K., Gaba, D. M., & Howard, S. K. (2006). So many roads: Facilitated debriefing in healthcare. *Simulation in Healthcare, 1*(1), 23–25.

Fanning, R. M., & Gaba, D. M. (2007). The role of debriefing in simulation-based learning. *Simulation in Healthcare, 2*(2), 115–125. doi:10.1097/SIH.0b013e3180315539

Flanagan, B. (2008). Debriefing: Theory and practice. In R. H. Riley (Ed.), *Manual of simulation in healthcare* (pp. 155–170). New York, NY: Oxford University Press.

Flin, R., Patey, R., Glavin, R., & Maran, N. (2010). Anaesthetists' non-technical skills. *British Journal of Anaesthesia, 105*(1), 38–44. doi:10.1093/bja/aeq134

Foa, E. B. (2010). Psychological debriefing for adults. In F. E. e. al (Ed.), *Effective treatments for PTSD* (2nd ed., pp. 539–541). New York, NY: Guilford Press.

Gaba, D. M. (2004). The future vision of simulation in health care. *Qual Saf Health Care, 13*(Suppl. 1), i2–10. doi:10.1136/qhc.13.suppl_1.i2

Gaba, H. S., Fish, K. J., Smith, B. E., & Sowb, Y. A. (2001). Simulation-based training in anesthesia crisis resource management (ACRM): A decade of experience. *Simulation and Gaming, 32*(2), 175–193.

Gibbs, G. (1988). *Learning by doing: A guide to teaching and learning methods*. Oxford: Further Educational Unit, Oxford Polytechnic.

Hart, D., McNeil, M. A., Griswold-Theodorson, S., Bhatia, K., & Joing, S. (2012). High fidelity case-based simulation debriefing: Everything you need to know. *Academic Emergency Medicine, 19*(9), E1084. doi:10.1111/j.1553-2712.2012.01423.x

Howard, S. K., Gaba, D. M., Fish, K. J., Yang, G., & Sarnquist, F. H. (1992). Anesthesia crisis resource management training: Teaching anesthesiologists to handle critical incidents. *Aviation, Space, and Environmental Medicine, 63*(9), 763–770.

Issenberg, S. B., McGaghie, W. C., Petrusa, E. R., Lee Gordon, D., & Scalese, R. J. (2005). Features and uses of high-fidelity medical simulations that lead to effective learning: A BEME systematic review. *Medical Teacher, 27*(1), 10–28. doi:10.1080/01421590500046924

Kelly, J. (2006). An overview of conflict. *Dimensions of Critical Care Nursing, 25*(1), 22–28.

Kolb, D. A. (1984). *Experiential learning : Experience as the source of learning and development.* Englewood Cliffs, NJ: Prentice-Hall.

Lederman, L. (1992). Debriefing: Toward a systematic assessment of theory and practice. *Simulation and Gaming, 23*(2), 145–160.

Leever, A. M., Hulst, M. V., Berendsen, A. J., Boendemaker, P. M., Roodenburg, J. L., & Pols, J. (2010). Conflicts and conflict management in the collaboration between nurses and physicians – a qualitative study. *Journal of Interprofessional Care, 24*(6), 612–624. doi:10.3109/13561820903550762

McGaghie, W. C., Issenberg, S. B., Petrusa, E. R., & Scalese, R. J. (2010). A critical review of simulation-based medical education research: 2003–2009. *Medical Education, 44*(1), 50–63. doi:10.1111/j.1365-2923.2009.03547.x

Miller, G. E. (1990). The assessment of clinical skills/competence/performance. *Academic Medicine, 65*(9 Suppl.), S63–S67.

Mitchell, J. T. (1983). When disaster strikes . . . the critical incident stress debriefing process. *Journal of Emergency Medical Services, 8*, 36–39.

Murphy, R., Driscoll, P., & O'Driscoll, R. (2001). Emergency oxygen therapy for the COPD patient. *Emergency Medicine Journal, 18*(5), 333–339. doi:10.1136/emj.18.5.333

Overstreet, M. (2010). Ee-chats: The seven components of nursing debriefing. *Journal of Continuing Education in Nursing, 41*(12), 538–539. doi:10.3928/00220124-20101122-05

Owen, H., & Follows, V. (2006). GREAT simulation debriefing. *Medical Education, 40*(5), 488–489. doi:10.1111/j.1365-2929.2006.02421.x

Rater's Handbook—DASH. Retrieved from http://www.harvardmedsim.org/_media/DASH.handbook.2010.Final.Rev.2.pdf

Rosen, K. R. (2008). The history of medical simulation. *Journal of Critical Care, 23*(2), 157–166. doi:10.1016/j.jcrc.2007.12.004

Rubenfield, M., & Scheffer, B. (2005). *Crticial thinking tacts for nurses.* Sudbury MA: Jones and Bartlett.

Rudolph, J. W., Simon, R., Dufresne, R. L., & Raemer, D. B. (2006). There's no such thing as "nonjudgmental" debriefing: A theory and method for debriefing with good judgment. *Simulation in Healthcare, 1*(1), 49–55.

Rudolph, J. W., Simon, R., Raemer, D. B., & Eppich, W. J. (2008). Debriefing as formative assessment: Closing performance gaps in medical education. *Academic Emergency Medicine, 15*(11), 1010–1016. doi:10.1111/j.1553-2712.2008.00248.x

Salas, E., Klein, C., King, H., Salisbury, M., Augenstein, J. S., Birnbach, D. J., . . . Upshaw, C. (2008). Debriefing medical teams: 12 evidence-based best practices and tips. *Joint Commission Journal on Quality and Patient Safety, 34*(9), 518–527.

Salas, E., Wilson, K. A., Burke, C. S., & Priest, H. A. (2005). Using simulation-based training to improve patient safety: What does it take? *Joint Commission Journal on Quality and Patient Safety, 31*(7), 363–371.

Savoldelli, G. L., Naik, V. N., Park, J., Joo, H. S., Chow, R., & Hamstra, S. J. (2006). Value of debriefing during simulated crisis management: Oral versus video-assisted oral feedback. *Anesthesiology, 105*(2), 279–285.

Sawyer, T., Sierocka-Castaneda, A., Chan, D., Berg, B., Lustik, M., & Thompson, M. (2012). The effectiveness of video-assisted debriefing versus oral debriefing alone at improving neonatal resuscitation performance: A randomized trial. *Simulation in Healthcare, 7*(4), 213–221. doi:10.1097/SIH.0b013e3182578eae

Scherer, L. A., Chang, M. C., Meredith, J. W., & Battistella, F. D. (2003). Videotape review leads to rapid and sustained learning. *American Journal of Surgery, 185*(6), 516–520.

Schön, D. A. (1983). *The reflective practitioner: How professionals think in action.* New York, NY: Basic Books.

Simon, R., Raemer, D. B., & Rudolph, J. W. (2009). *Debriefing assessment for simulation in healthcare.* Retrieved from http://www.harvardmedsim.org/debriefing-assesment-simulation-healthcare.php

Walsh, M. (2011). Narrative pedagogy and simulation: Future directions for nursing education. *Nurse Education in Practice, 11*(3), 216–219. doi:10.1016/j.nepr.2010.10.006

M. Isabel Friedman
Martin Doerfler
Michal Tamuz

3: Safety Hub: Research and Role of a Simulation Center in a System-Wide Initiative to Reduce Sepsis

In accord with a health system's extensive campaign to increase awareness, improve treatment, and reduce mortality due to sepsis, simulation plays a pivotal role as one in a series of educational measures that target critical care and emergency nurses. Their vital role as frontline caretakers makes it imperative that they are fully familiar with the standard definitions and clinical presentation of sepsis and can practice according to evidence-based management guidelines. Significantly improved metrics attributable to early recognition and management of severe sepsis and septic shock support the concept of systems integration—a fourth domain of simulation, in addition to education, assessment, and research.

Simulation improves performance in the clinical context, facilitating the acquisition and application of cognitive, behavioral, psychomotor, and interprofessional skills. It directly impacts individuals and teams by providing the instrumentality for perceiving and remediating errors and knowledge gaps of all kinds. However, in addition, conceived as a strategic tool of systems engineering, simulation may also be directly and purposefully integrated with broader initiatives that involve clinical research (McGaghie, Draycott, Dunn, Lopez, & Stefanidis, 2011). It is a versatile tool that can serve clinical practice and crisis management, in brief, in ways that are more effective than didactic educational methods alone. Using simulation to institutionalize specific evidence-based guidelines and protocols across an entire health care system is one of its most valuable features. The problem of life-threatening sepsis and septic shock, currently of epidemic proportion and cause for an ongoing and worldwide health initiative, is an instructive example.

Sepsis: The Major Challenge

As with heart attack and stroke, the onset of severe sepsis represents a distinct challenge in terms of vigilance, critical thinking, patient evaluation, and time to treatment. Severe sepsis strikes about 750,000 persons each year in North America and kills an estimated 200,000—more deaths than from breast cancer, prostate cancer, and HIV/AIDS combined (Czura, 2010). As the leading cause of death in noncardiac intensive care units (ICUs), severe sepsis counts for about one in five of all admissions to ICUs.

Defined as acute organ dysfunction or tissue hypoperfusion secondary to infection, sepsis is not a unitary disease but a syndrome that represents a potentially life-threatening immune response (Edwards, 1993; Schorr, Zanotti, & Dellinger, 2013). Recognition can be difficult. By appearance, its onset may be insidious, masked by other conditions, and unpredictable. A patient presenting with two of the criteria for systemic inflammatory response syndrome (SIRS) plus a known or suspected infection should be categorized as having sepsis. Severe sepsis and septic shock comprise the acute emergency phases of a fourfold spectrum that begins with SIRS and can progress to sepsis (Balk, 2013). Time to treatment is a major factor, with early diagnosis crucial.

Current efforts to raise awareness and reduce mortality from severe sepsis and septic shock date to the Surviving Sepsis Campaign (SSC), a performance-improvement initiative that first took shape in 2002 (Levy et al., 2010). A consortium of three organizations (European Society of Intensive Care Medicine, Society of Critical Care Medicine, and International Sepsis Forum) developed a registry and management guidelines for care, first published in 2004 (Dellinger et al., 2004). Based on accumulated data that showed early identification should be able to reduce mortality, the guidelines were comprised of treatment goals, known as "bundles," to be initiated over specific time frames in response to identification and staging. As an evidence-based set of critical procedures, the Sepsis 3-Hour Bundle and Sepsis 6-Hour Bundle are more rigorous and demanding than a simple checklist and carry a higher level of individual and team accountability. The initial clinical goal of SSC, when the guidelines were published in 2004, was to reduce mortality from severe sepsis and septic shock by 25% within 5 years. In fact, an updated version, published in 2008, signaled modest, documented success with compliance, including a drop in mortality (5.4%) over the first 2 years and reflected the assessment that "the data are encouraging and supportive of the Campaign's creating beneficial effects both on patient care and patient outcome" (Levy et al., 2010, p. 228). The most recent revision of the guidelines, published in 2013, represents an advance in terms of consensus: their final formulation owes to a committee of 68 international experts associated with 30 international organizations (Dellinger et al., 2013; Kleinpell, Aitken, & Schorr, 2013). But it should be added that several components of the SSC guidelines remain nondefinitive and under continued scrutiny; they represent a work-in-progress (Barochia, Cui, & Eichacker, 2013).

As has been the case with other life-threatening emergencies, progress to combat severe sepsis has not proved to be either simple or straightforward. Throughout the world, public awareness of sepsis is low (Rubulotta et al., 2009) and adoption of the guidelines by hospitals has been relatively slow (Dellinger et al., 2008). The developers themselves recognized that the "publication of guidelines often do not lead to changes in clinical behavior and guidelines are rarely, if ever, integrated into bedside practice in a timely fashion." How to best achieve knowledge transfer has remained, in effect, "an unanswered question" (Levy et al., 2010, p. 223). By themselves the SSC guidelines suggest or point to the detailed ways by which health systems can apply them to improve outcomes in clinical practice: "Ultimately, hospital-based efforts and local protocol development [are] the purview of individual improvement teams at each institution or network" (Levy et al., 2010, p. 224).

Implementation: Adapting the Guidelines

The North Shore-LIJ Health System (NS-LIJ) adapted the SSC guidelines and implemented a program to reduce sepsis mortality in 2008, with a decision by its president and CEO, Michael J. Dowling, as part of a broader effort to stem preventable deaths. With 15 hospitals, including 5 tertiary facilities, counting more than 600,000 emergency visits annually, NS-LIJ had developed as a single-governance entity with a unitary management and research institute capable of formulating performance metrics and tracking sepsis-related data through the entire system. In fact, an early retrospective census showed that the number of deaths from severe sepsis and septic shock were higher than expected and ranked as the top All Patient Refined Diagnosis Related Group (APR-DRG) and represented the system's highest single cause of in-hospital mortality.

Although a detailed account of the system-wide evaluation by the NS-LIJ Sepsis Task Force lies beyond the scope of this chapter, it resulted in the formulation of multiple goals while exploring the effectiveness of alternative solutions in each of the health system facilities. Importantly, subsequent implementation of the SSC guidelines was specific to each facility and addressed special challenges with respect to emergency departments and medical–surgical units. The Task Force's experience in refining and shaping the guidelines reflected, more broadly, the fact that severe sepsis and sepsis shock are fairly simple to define, but identifying the patients who are potential victims of severe sepsis is by no means straightforward. Invasive procedures may be required for both evaluation and monitoring and there is no "gold standard" marker for the disease; diagnosis is by consensus and relies on the lowest level of evidence. Implementation of the clinical guidelines was necessarily accompanied by a series of educational efforts to ensure clinical understanding of the disease and its physiology, the algorithm and screening tool, the severe sepsis "bundles," and data collection materials for monitoring compliance.

The corporate strategy to reduce sepsis mortality resulted in a partnership with the Institute for Healthcare Improvement (IHI), a nonprofit group that helps to structure innovation in health care (www.ihi.org/Pages/default.aspx). Their collaborative input with clinical researchers at NS-LIJ resulted in more fully developed strategies for implementation and data tracking (Resar, Griffin, Haraden, & Nolan, 2012).

Implications for Nursing

With early recognition regarded as key to successful outcomes, the role for emergency department and critical care nurses was understood, though not always explicitly, as crucial to initiation of the sepsis bundles. Prompt identification of signs and symptoms—ideally, as with stroke and myocardial infarction, within the "golden hour" (1 hour within onset of hypotension)—is viewed as key to mortality reduction; at that juncture there exists an approximately 6-hour window of opportunity in terms of treatment (Dellinger et al., 2004; Gross, 2006). Every hour of delay has been associated with a 7.6% increased risk of death (Kumar et al., 2006). Although the system-wide initiation of educational programs at NS-LIJ intended to reach physicians and nurses alike with comprehensive information, a targeted education program for emergency department and critical care nurses was a clear objective.

From an interprofessional and adult learning standpoint, investing critical care and emergency nurses with the comprehensive knowledge base and recommendations of the SSC would require more than didactic presentations. As early as 2007, research using simulation as an evaluative tool had indicated "great heterogeneity in the performance of both interns and whole teams" in sepsis management (Ottestad, Boulet, & Lighthall, 2007, p. 769). A series of studies with simulated patients showed that "[l]eadership, communication and anticipation all play a role in defining the adequacy of group performance" (Ottestad et al., p. 773). The Stanford researchers, in their series of 23 sepsis scenarios, noted that the team with the lowest technical score also had the lowest nontechnical score—a case study, they suggested, of how ineffective leadership could result in chaotic management that neutralizes the effectiveness of otherwise competent practitioners.

Taming Sepsis Education Program

The Taming Sepsis Education Program (TSEP),[1] inaugurated in 2012, aims to provide registered nurses in emergency departments and critical care units at NS-LIJ with a comprehensive educational program to ensure they recognize SIRS and all symptoms and signs of sepsis, severe sepsis, and septic shock. The program employs two learning modalities that are thematically integrated: a didactic portion with web-based curricula, and clinical practice using simulation.

Didactic Learning Four learning modules comprise the didactic portion of TSEP. Nurses complete each module online and progress to the next only after successfully passing a posttest. The first three modules are essentially preparatory to the clinical content and involve both new knowledge and review. Participants begin by taking the on-line course based on IHI "bundles"—defined as a small number of evidence-based interventions for a specific patient population in a particular setting. The concept is not familiar to all and the bundles module provides the necessary definitions, explains the importance of bundles, distinguishes them by contrast with checklist protocols, and discusses the limitations of their use.

Two more courses in TSEP further prepare nurses for the course in sepsis management. A refresher course in communications, teamwork, and the various concepts associated with Team Strategies and Tools to Enhance Performance and Patient Safety (Team-STEPPS®) is one. For a life-threatening condition such as sepsis, nurses need to practice the Situation, Background, Assessment, and Recommendation (SBAR) technique, used to provide requests and recommendations succinctly and systematically. They must also know how to employ the Two-Challenge Rule if their concerns are not met in a timely way. In addition, nurses also follow a web-based program aligned with the Culturally Linguistically Appropriate Services (CLAS) standards (Diamond, Wilson-Stronks, & Jacobs, 2010; Messias, 2003). The catchment area served by NS-LIJ includes one of the most culturally diverse populations in the world; the borough of Queens alone is populated by residents of more than 100 nationalities who speak some 167 languages.

The final module in the didactic modality is the comprehensive brief course on the signs, symptoms, and stages of sepsis, as well as thought-provoking case studies. This peer-reviewed continuing education offering was developed by nurse leaders and educators at NS-LIJ who were members of the Sepsis Task Force. Learners are introduced to the distinguishing features of SIRS, sepsis, severe sepsis, and septic shock; they are provided the most current and context-relevant information on how to assess patients and how to discuss their assessment findings concerning patients at increased risk for sepsis. They review the signs and symptoms of tissue hypoxia and organ dysfunction; they learn the current recommendations for fluid resuscitation, and, more generally, the rationale for the various treatments for septic shock.

"Putting it all Together" Through Simulation All nurses who take part in TSEP participate in high-fidelity simulation scenarios that require critical thinking and decision making in the context of clinical emergencies that involve SIRS, sepsis, severe sepsis, or septic shock. Participants also include physicians and/or nurse practitioners. Drawing upon the clinical examples used in the didactic portion of the program, content experts developed scenarios that cover sepsis as it might appear in patients with pneumonia or postoperation infection in hip replacement, severe sepsis as it might appear in a patient with cellulitis of the leg or narcotic drug overdose, and septic shock in the context of urinary tract infection.[2]

Case Example: Postoperative Hip Infection The nurse participant, informed only that the patient is a 47-year-old woman recovering from hip surgery, enters the hospital room to discover the patient complaining of pain at the surgical site.[3] Examining the site, the nurse finds it is inflamed, warm to the touch, and purulent. The patient's pulse is elevated and her respirations are 22 breaths per minute.

The task of the nurse participant, recognizing sepsis, is to translate into action the knowledge and skills acquired or reviewed in the didactic portion of the program. In the case at hand, she should now contact the attending physician or nurse practitioner and provide a concise description of the patient, her assessment that the patient is now exhibiting signs and symptoms of sepsis, and make the entire series of necessary requests: two blood cultures, a complete blood count, an electrolyte panel, and an order for a lactate level. The nurse signals her recommendation to start an intravenous (IV) line and provide acetaminophen for elevated temperature; she suggests a maintenance dose of fluids and requests an antibiotic.

When a nurse practitioner, physician's assistant, or physician is available to participate in sepsis simulations, the genuine interprofessional interaction augments to the realism of the experience and further enriches the debriefing session, with a view to enhanced collaboration and teamwork.

Extensive debriefing follows the simulation, which has been video recorded so that key portions can be replayed to underscore any issues around performance. Debriefs are wide ranging and may cover the underlying scientific knowledge base, issues of medication, teamwork, and all recommendations. Scenarios may be readily adapted for cases to take place in the critical care unit, emergency department, or on the medical–surgical floor. Their aim is to consolidate learning, reinforce skills, and serve as a check on performance that confirms or disconfirms individual success with TSEP.

Metrics and Evaluation

We recovered the raw sepsis, severe sepsis, and septic shock mortality data for the entire NS-LIJ, from 2008 through 2013. As Figure 3.1 indicates, we noted several landmarks: issuance of the Sepsis Task Force Guidelines (February 2009), a new focus on timely administration of antibiotics in emergency departments (March 2011), and initiation of quality improvement projects (April 2013). TSEP was inaugurated in 2012, and by 2014 more than 1,100 critical care nurses had both completed the didactic portion and participated in clinical simulations.

A review of the data (see Figure 3.1) shows a broadly gradual, sustained downturn in mortality rates from sepsis, cumulative to a 50% reduction in NS-LIJ hospitals over the course of 4 years, from 31% in 2009 to 15% in October 2013. Although the data do not permit analysis of the specific impact of TSEP, the program was not designed as a stand-alone initiative. It should instead be considered as part of the broader strategic effort both to reduce mortality from sepsis and to improve patient safety throughout the health system. The collaboration initiative targets all forms of sepsis. It focuses on early recognition,

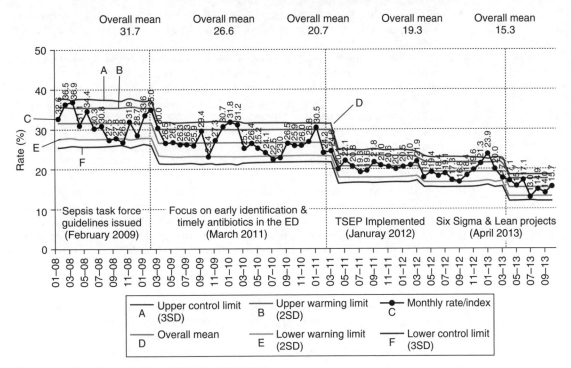

Figure 3.1 Sepsis mortality at NS-LIJ, 2008–2013.

prompt collection of blood cultures, and urgent administration of antibiotics; it seeks to improve processes with respect to appropriately timed lactate levels and rapid and adequate fluid administration. Simulation as an integral part of this system-wide initiative represents its use in the context of formulating and achieving strategic goals. Its courses and curricula are designed in conjunction with the tools of systems engineering to improve clinical outcomes with lasting organizational impact. It represents, in short, a multipronged effort to build a culture of patient safety.

NOTES

1. The Taming Sepsis Educational Program for Registered Nurses (TSEP) was supported by funds from the Division of Nursing (DN), Bureau of Health Professions (BHPr), Health Resources and Services Administration (HRSA), and Department of Health and Human Services (DHHS) under grant award #1 D11HP22203 (NEPQR HRSA – 11-041).
2. When the TSEP program was extended to include pediatric nurses, topics also included cold shock in a case of gastroenteritis, normotensive shock in acute myeloid leukemia, and warm shock in pneumonia.
3. Moulage applied to the computerized manikin simulates the appearance of the infection; the patient's words and any necessary further descriptive expressions are supplied by the simulation facilitator.

REFERENCES

Balk, R. A. (2013). Systemic inflammatory response syndrome (SIRS): Where did it come from and is it still relevant today? *Virulence, 5*(1), 20–26.

Barochia, A. V., Cui, X., & Eichacker, P. Q. (2013). The surviving sepsis campaign's revised sepsis bundles. *Current Infectious Disease Report, 15*(5), 385–393. doi:10.1007/s11908-013-0351-3

Czura, C. J. (2010). Merinoff symposium 2010: Sepsis—an international call to action. *Molecular Medicine, 16*(5–6), 157–158. doi:10.2119/molmed.2010.00001.editorial

Dellinger, R. P., Carlet, J. M., Masur, H., Gerlach, H., Calandra, T., Cohen, J., . . . Levy, M. M. (2004). Surviving sepsis campaign guidelines for management of severe sepsis and septic shock. *Critical Care Medicine, 32*(3), 858–873.

Dellinger, R. P., Levy, M. M., Carlet, J. M., Bion, J., Parker, M. M., Jaeschke, R., . . . Critical Care, M. (2008). Surviving sepsis campaign: International guidelines for management of severe sepsis and septic shock: 2008. *Critical Care Medicine, 36*(1), 296–327. doi:10.1097/01.ccm.0000298158.12101.41

Dellinger, R. P., Levy, M., Rhodes, A., Annane, D., Gerlach, H., Opal, S., . . . Moreno, R. (2013). Surviving sepsis campaign: International guidelines for management of severe sepsis and septic shock, 2012. *Intensive Care Med, 39*(2), 165–228. doi:10.1007/s00134-012-2769-8

Diamond, L. C., Wilson-Stronks, A., & Jacobs, E. A. (2010). Do hospitals measure up to the national culturally and linguistically appropriate services standards? *Medical care, 48*(12), 1080–1087. doi:10.1097/MLR.0b013e3181f380bc

Edwards, J. D. (1993). Management of septic shock. *British Medical Journals, 306*(6893), 1661–1664.

Gross, P. A. (2006). Hypotension and mortality in septic shock: The "golden hour". *Critical Care Medicine, 34*(6), 1819–1820. doi:10.1097/01.ccm.0000220054.95214.7d

Kleinpell, R., Aitken, L., & Schorr, C. A. (2013). Implications of the new international sepsis guidelines for nursing care. *American Journal of Critical Care, 22*(3), 212–222. doi:10.4037/ajcc2013158

Kumar, A., Haery, C., Paladugu, B., Kumar, A., Symeonides, S., Taiberg, L., . . . Parrillo, J. E. (2006). The duration of hypotension before the initiation of antibiotic treatment is a critical determinant of survival in a murine model of Escherichia coli septic shock: Association with serum lactate and inflammatory cytokine levels. *Journal of Infectious Diseases, 193*(2), 251–258. doi:10.1086/498909

Levy, M. M., Dellinger, R. P., Townsend, S. R., Linde-Zwirble, W. T., Marshall, J. C., Bion, J., . . . Angus, D. C. (2010). The Surviving Sepsis Campaign: Results of an international guideline-based performance improvement program targeting severe sepsis. *Intensive Care Medicine, 36*(2), 222–231. doi:10.1007/s00134-009-1738-3

McGaghie, W. C., Draycott, T. J., Dunn, W. F., Lopez, C. M., & Stefanidis, D. (2011). Evaluating the impact of simulation on translational patient outcomes. *Simulation in Healthcare, 6*(Suppl.), S42–S47. doi:10.1097/SIH.0b013e318222fde9

Messias, D. K. (2003). What nurses need to know about the National Standards for Culturally and Linguistically Appropriate Services (CLAS) in health care. *South Carolina Nurse, 10*(3), 23–24.

Ottestad, E., Boulet, J. R., & Lighthall, G. K. (2007). Evaluating the management of septic shock using patient simulation. *Critical Care Medicine, 35*(3), 769–775. doi:10.1097/01.ccm.0000256849.75799.20

Resar, R., Griffin, F., Haraden, C., & Nolan, T. (2012). *Using Care Bundles to Improve Health Care Quality IHI Innovation Series white paper*. Cambridge, MA: Institute for Healthcare Improvement.

Rubulotta, F. M., Ramsay, G., Parker, M. M., Dellinger, R. P., Levy, M. M., & Poeze, M. (2009). An international survey: Public awareness and perception of sepsis. *Critical Care Medicine, 37*(1), 167–170.

Schorr, C. A., Zanotti, S., & Dellinger, R. P. (2013). Severe sepsis and septic shock: Management and performance improvement. *Virulence, 5*(1), 190–199.

Two: Adult Interprofessional Teams

Alan R. Hartman
Stephen Bello
Kristen Rojas
Robert L. Kerner Jr.
Ronald Ulrich

4: Safety From the Outset: Creating an Interprofessional Team in a Cardiothoracic Intensive Care Unit

*An open heart cardiac surgical care unit, established over the course of a brief
4.5-month startup schedule, made extensive use of realistic high-fidelity simulation and principles of interprofessional learning to create a tertiary care
program in a community hospital acquired by a nonprofit health system with
all requisite and maximum attention to patient safety. Knowledge acquired
through simulation at the Patient Safety Institute continues to help organize
further teamwork improvements, including revised protocol for the handoff
of patients from the operating room (OR) to the cardiothoracic intensive care
unit (CT-ICU).*

Cardiothoracic intensive care units (CT-ICUs) have evolved in conjunction with
cardiac surgery over the course of nearly half a century and currently embody a
host of advances in the surveillance and treatment of heart patients after surgical intervention. Today, typical core teams in the CT-ICU include critical care
nurses, intensivists, perfusionists, respiratory therapists, physician assistants,
and staff nurses. Their surveillance of patients in concert with surgeons and

anesthesiologists in the hours after surgery and during the dynamic phase of recovery involves minute-by-minute assessment and constant readiness to intervene. Although mortality in the course of open heart surgery is low, the risk of complications in the hours and sometimes days after surgery remains relatively high. In addition to the whole panoply of comorbidities, potential problems include bleeding, arrhythmia, renal failure, low cardiac index, cardiogenic shock, a variety of neurological issues, and gastrointestinal dysfunction.

With the expansion of monitoring technologies and available interventions, together with a growing number of reoperative surgeries in fragile patients, CT-ICUs benefit from nurses and allied staff who operate as interprofessional teams that are largely free of the top-down hierarchical system of authority that individuals may bring to the unit, owing to background and education. It is worth remembering that not long ago, for example, there existed a commonly accepted distinction between nursing and "practicing medicine" in intensive care units (Roth & Daze, 1984). The nurse would initiate treatment based on "assessment of the patient's symptoms; not through making differential medical diagnosis" (Coombs, 2003). Today, however, the nature of much intensive care blurs or eliminates that distinction and, more generally, "it should be recognized that all members of the multidisciplinary team are crucial to patient care and outcome"(Smith, 1998).

From the Ground Up

The administrative decision to create a new Department of Cardiovascular and Thoracic Surgery at Southside Hospital owed to both local demographics and to the prospect of improving service after the hospital was incorporated into North Shore-LIJ (NS-LIJ), a large nonprofit health system. Southside serves Suffolk County on Long Island, New York, one of the largest and most populous counties in the nation. The county is largely middle class and urban, with a population of 1.5 million, including some 210,000 residents age 65 or older (Bureau, 2012).

At the time of acquisition, however, Southside was not a tertiary care facility. Surgeons at only one hospital in Suffolk County performed open heart procedures and its location for most county residents was not central. Of patients undergoing cardiac surgery at NS-LIJ system-wide, about 30% were Suffolk County residents. In 2009 system administrators submitted a revised Certificate of Need to New York State health authorities that included a proposal to open a comprehensive open heart surgery program at Southside; in mid-September 2010 the Department of Health (DOH) ruled in favor of the new unit.

Plans to open a state-of-the-art cardiothoracic surgery department in a former community hospital obviously meant changes in infrastructure and organization. With respect to the CT-ICU, two features were of special significance. First, we decided against any sort of "acclimation period" during which we would accept or reroute patients based on severity of disease or the specific intervention required. We would not reject patients who were eligible for heart surgery, including older patients and cases calling for repeat bypass or other more complex procedures. This decision reflected our view that the new campus at Southside was in fact an extension of the existing program at NS-LIJ and would employ surgeons and anesthesiologists experienced in that program.

In addition, our plan called for opening the program within 4.5 months of approval, a highly accelerated time frame. Normally, such a process could be expected to take 12 to 18 months. To meet the challenges imposed by the startup date and the plan to open a fully functioning program, we made extensive use of the Center for Learning and Innovation (CLI) and its allied Patient Safety Institute (PSI).

Simulation Used Strategically

We were aware that creating a CT-ICU offered the opportunity to ensure development of a culture of safety consonant with the current national patient safety movement. We also had previously used simulation at other CT-ICU units in the NS-LIJ system, turning to the PSI to enhance communications skills and raise the comfort level of personnel. At North Shore University Hospital, our monthly simulation training for all personnel had demonstrated to our satisfaction the value of team building. With time-to-open on an accelerated schedule, the necessity of educating an entire new team for Southside encouraged us to look to PSI and plan extensive use of simulation.

Transparency and metrics would provide useful, suggestive confirmation of overall success of the new program. As we discuss further in the following, New York State has for more than 2 decades provided rigorous hospital-level data concerning short-term mortality and complications from cardiac surgery (Hannan, Cozzens, King, Walford, & Shah, 2012). These statistics are published annually and are publically available. They offer, in effect, a built-in measure of the success or failure of any cardiothoracic surgery program in New York State and represent a performance yardstick for programs elsewhere.

Building an Interprofessional Team

Simulation for team training and patient safety did not take place in a context removed from the day-to-day development of the new program. Indeed, opening the CT-ICU put Southside Hospital's integration into the larger health system to a test. It required the addition of about 70 employees, including several dozen nurses. We hired intensivists, perfusionists, physician assistants, nurse practitioners, laboratory technicians, respiratory therapists, and administrative personnel. We purchased equipment and prepared a suite of two new operating rooms while upgrading the existing ICU. We were tasked, in brief, with creating new infrastructure while ensuring everyone possessed the requisite competencies in a physical plant where those competencies did not yet exist and when details as to procedures were yet to be determined.

Orientation of staff, as a practical matter, naturally involved a didactic component. For the CT-ICU nursing staff, for example, we required all RNs undergo a critical care challenge assessment and complete the Essentials of Critical Care Orientation (ECCO) developed by the American Association of Critical-Care Nurses. A 3-day orientation course for experienced ICU nurses included an overview of procedures and postoperative care, reviews of cardiothoracic surgery, hemodynamics, bedside monitor operations and cardiac devices, the Surgical Care Improvement Project (SCIP) protocols, code blue procedures, and ICU flow sheet documentation. Wherever possible, based in part on our past experience with CLI/PSI, we employed principles of interdisciplinary team building. In general, our recruitment and orientation efforts reflected awareness that, for an ICU, high staff turnover threatens to disrupt patient care and adversely affect quality of care (Friedman, Cooper, Click, & Fitzpatrick, 2011; Shortell et al., 1994).

All such day-to-day efforts and initiatives in the days and weeks leading up to inauguration of the CT-ICU in February 2011 constituted the larger background and context for a series of simulation exercises designed to ensure highest standards of patient safety. Their goals were to positively impact interactive behavior, refine cognitive and motor skills, and improve situational awareness. A retrospective analysis suggests that simulation facilitated team learning in four major areas of activity: (i) regularization of language and coordination of behavior, (ii) reduction of the authority gradient, (iii) group acclimation to schedule and equipment, and (iv) interprofessional team building and problem solving.

Regularizing Team Language and Complementary Skill Sets

Patients in the immediate aftermath of open heart surgery are not only intensively monitored but they are surrounded by a constant stream of purpose-driven language and action. Our protocols, for example, consider that CT-ICU handoff begins about 30 minutes before the end of surgery with a telephone call from the OR that provides basic details about the patient and procedure. The surgeon, anesthesiologist, and physician assistant transport the patient to the unit and remain at the bedside until a fully detailed handoff is complete and thoroughly understood by the entire team. Signout can take 20 minutes or longer and includes detailed past history, pertinent events concerning the procedure just completed, what may be expected in the next several hours, and the game plan for the rest of the day. There is also a written report in a prepared format. Each morning there is a multidisciplinary report out on every patient in the cardiothoracic service, which is led by the physician assistant who cared for the patients overnight. All aspects of care are open for discussion and participants include the surgeon, nurses, the pharmacist, physical therapist, social worker, and dietician.

CT-ICU teams must employ a common language for their protocols and procedures to work seamlessly (Manojlovich, 2010). In an established unit, acculturation of a newly hired nurse or other provider is straightforward, with orientation and adjustment to an existing set of algorithms with associated terminology. But our unique situation brought to the CT-ICU an entire staff of newly hired critical care nurses, all experienced but with varied capabilities and recruited from different health systems and hospitals. Similar issues arose with physician assistants, nurse practitioners, and other staff. In brief, everyone possessed the underlying skill set involved in postoperative care of cardiac patients, but they did not know each other or speak the same technical language.

Although didactic instruction and orientation could be expected to help regularize language, it could not hope to do so to the extent required in the time available. Development of a common language and a shared mental model became a common theme in simulation at PSI. The nursing director and nurse manager would choose groups to attend day-long sessions and explicitly compose them so they included people who did not know one another. Multidisciplinary teams, numbering 6 to 10, would carry out simulations in a fully equipped mock ICU at the PSI, observed from the control room and video recorded; debriefings took place in a relaxed setting in a separate room. A first day of simulations was followed by a second day during which one of the unit's surgeons was present as an observer and active in the debriefings.

The simulations helped resolve language and skill discrepancies. Nurses from one background, for example, referred to bypass surgeries by the common term "cabbages"; those from another hospital simply abbreviated CABG as "C." Use of these terms with reference to repeat surgery could cause further confusion: "Cabbage-times-three" and "C-3" both referred to a patient undergoing a triple bypass operation. Some nurses referred to the "O-two sensor" and others referred to it with the proprietary name of the sensor manufacturer. Problems of language extended to communication that could be verbal or written: "Mitral valve repair" on a report might appear as "MVr," only to be misinterpreted as "mitral valve *replacement*," a much different procedure.

Simulation also helped to detect nonverbal cues and "private language" problems that could cause confusion. Several nurses recruited from the same hospital had developed a gestural language among themselves. One nurse would say to another: "I need one of those ____" and by a hand gesture her interlocutor would immediately respond with "I'll get it," leaving the rest of the team out of the communication loop.

Eliminating an Authority Gradient

Rigid hierarchy embedded in the tradition and training of most caregivers can contribute to lapses in patient safety through interference with communication across grades of authority (Cosby & Croskerry, 2004). A specific recommendation in *To Err Is Human* counsels careful error reporting without reprisals, using "simulation whenever possible" and developing "a working culture in which communication flows freely regardless of authority gradient" (Kohn, Corrigan, & Donaldson, 2000). With respect to ICUs, one classic concurrent incident research study of a medical–surgical ICU documented a high rate of reported errors that was in great part attributed to faulty communication between physicians and nurses (Donchin et al., 1995). Despite widespread agreement that hierarchy should be deemphasized and interprofessional teams encouraged, we could reasonably expect that issues associated with communication and the authority gradient would arise in creating and managing a new CT-ICU. So they did.

Simulation offers a physical setting for observing errors in communication and at the same time provides a safe environment for people to open up and discuss issues of patient care and communication. Conflicts associated with retentions of hierarchy, which are out of place in interprofessional teams, can be exposed, discussed, and worked through. "[C]reating a safe atmosphere where team members feel they can speak up if they have any safety concerns or issues with the quality of care provided patients is essential" (Reader, Flin, Mearns, & Cuthbertson, 2007).

Our simulation of a pneumothorax due to ruptured bleb, with a group of nurses and physician assistants, provided a striking example. Burt Hogg, as the patient was known—represented by a SimMan—called the nurse into the room after he began suffering from shortness of breath. In order to represent a case of anterior pneumothorax, the patient's right-side breath sounds were diminished but not absent. Upon diagnosis, the nursing staff was to assist and assemble the chest drainage device. If all steps were taken in a timely fashion, the patient would improve. If not, Mr. Hogg could progress to respiratory failure.

During one session with this scenario, participants failed to rapidly recognize what was wrong with the patient. The session was stressful and the surgeon, observing from the control room, felt frustrated, but he followed the advice of the CT-ICU director and let the simulation play out. During the subsequent debriefing, one nurse stated: "I knew it was pneumothorax; I had a feeling it was." Asked why she kept silent, she replied: "Nurses don't diagnose."

Here the surgeon addressed the multidisciplinary group: "But I want you to say whatever you're thinking. I'm here as the chairman to tell you that I don't want you ever to worry about being wrong. You're excellent clinicians and if your assessment tells you the patient is sick, I need you to tell me that he's getting sick, not call me an hour later and tell me: 'He's been sick and now we're certain that he's dying.' I want you to pull the trigger early. Take ownership of the problem and take action. Treat the patient. Put the needle in the patient's chest. Then call me about the good work done."

This extemporaneous response emphasized both teamwork in a crisis and the wider focus of interprofessional team behavior. Taking place in the fundamentally inquisitive context of debriefing, it worked as a cutaway illustration of how to neutralize the hierarchy gradient. Issues of "power and conflict" have been repeatedly documented, specifically with respect to ICUs (Coombs, 2003; Shortell et al., 1994; Thomas, Sexton, & Helmreich, 2003). In general, some level of hierarchy or authority gradient is best considered, at present and in the near future, to be a problematic constant in any CT-ICU. Older models of medical education, it may be assumed, have enduring effects on team culture and competencies.

Team Learning With Complex Scenarios: Communication and Coordination

Communication failures are at the root of approximately 7 in 10 sentinel events, according to a 2006 report by The Joint Commission (Salas, DiazGranados, Weaver, & King, 2008). We wanted to test how our CT-ICU team would respond to interference with customary communications when they involved, for example, family members during crises. Could the team continue to communicate professionally and rapidly adapt to unexpected events that were best met with a request for more help or required the team itself to subdivide? Could the team deal adequately with distractions? Could members avoid multitasking with the risk of losing focus on the patient?

We developed a scenario—more or less spontaneously—that was similar to the pneumothorax presented above but with a set of complications. We employed a standardized patient (SP) to portray the patient's wife. She entered the hospital room during the crisis, posed questions and became obstreperous, started hyperventilating, and then fainted. In effect, she became a second patient and the team was compelled to treat her as well, choosing an ancillary leader who would install her in another room, where a second manikin took the place of the SP and had to be treated.

We also conducted simulations that tested competencies around machine malfunctions. Technologies that usually provide reliable information can generate perceptual dissonance and confusion when they fail for whatever reason, such that patient symptoms or behaviors do not match the output numbers. We designed scenarios that demonstrated how the patient's signs and symptoms should drive intervention in such cases and how to tell whether the machine output is faulty.

In-Situ Simulation and Handoff Improvements

Shortly before the program opened formally in February 2011, the site of simulation shifted from the Patient Safety Institute to the hospital itself. Brief simulation sessions followed by longer debriefings became a platform for orienting the staff to the unit's daily activities. A series of "dry runs" lasted a full week and included the OR staff in practicing the handoff procedure. Prior to opening, the staff worked together to develop efficiencies in transporting patients after surgery and in designing, organizing, and stocking the unit.

Group cohesion was an additional benefit of simulation learning. Over time it also helped bring about subsequent improvements as we recognized both individual instances of lost or faulty information transfer and a general impression that patient data were incomplete or not fully shared. In its initial form, our handoff procedure involved the anesthesiologist providing a postsurgery account and treatment details to the ICU team while the primary nurse was connecting the patient to monitoring equipment and a secondary nurse drew labs. As many as six or eight people could be gathered around the bedside, fostering confusion despite written reports. Working collectively, the nurses and physician assistants revised the process. Now the secondary nurse performs all monitoring hookup procedures during transfer while the primary nurse remains with the anesthesiologist at the foot of the bed, together with the surgeon and physician assistant. Instead of a linear narrative from the anesthesiologist, nurses have time to ask questions and ensure explicit language. The handoff is safer, quieter, more deliberate, and orderly. It is detailed oriented and complete, contributing to overall patient care.

Inauguration and Metrics

The Department of Cardiovascular and Thoracic Surgery at Southside Hospital opened in February 2011, a little more than 4 months after approval of the Certificate of Need. Over the next 13 months we performed open-heart surgery on 359 patients.

Ongoing data collection monitors the relative safety of cardiac surgery in New York State. Nearly a quarter century ago the DOH began to confront issues of hospital-level variations in heart surgery outcomes, and it succeeded in developing a biannual registry that continues to be published today, with the next report due in the fall of 2014.[1] By 1992 New York had the lowest risk-adjusted mortality of any state in the United States, and later editions of the registry document the striking improvement in mortality and morbidity rates for open-heart surgery. Hospitals are mandated to report both organization-wide and surgeon-specific outcomes on a rolling 3-year basis (Chen, Orav, & Epstein, 2012; Hannan et al., 2012). Past concern that some hospitals and surgeons might avoid taking high-risk patients was one component that helped us decide, in opening the program at Southside, to avoid any sort of acclimation period during which we rerouted such cases.

Statistics for our program, to be published in the 2014 report, will provide accurate and complete numbers for the various quality indicators dictated by the DOH, including overall 30-day mortality, stroke, myocardial infarction, deep sternal wound infection, gastrointestinal complications, renal failure, sepsis, respiratory failure, further surgery (resternotomy) for bleeding, or any unplanned return to the OR. In all these quality indicators, our data indicate that Southside Hospital will prove to have rates that are better or equal to accepted benchmark rates based on the most current DOH data. The 2014 report (in press) indicates that Southside was notable for being significantly below the state average for valve and valve/CABG risk-adjusted mortality and well within the acceptable range for CABGs.

These metrics, from our perspective, support an underlying message concerning patient safety. Our successful creation of a tertiary-level cardiac surgical care unit in a community hospital required planning and implementation that crucially incorporated strategies embedded in the concerted and organized use of high-fidelity simulation and the principles of interprofessional team building. Without them, the transformative accomplishment we describe here could not have happened.

NOTE

1. The most recent report, with statistics compiled for 2008-2010, was published in 2012. www.health.ny.gov/statistics/diseases/cardiovascular/heart_disease/docs/2008-2010_adult_cardiac_surgery.pdf

REFERENCES

Bureau, U. S. C. (2012). *Suffolk County*, New York. Retrieved from http://quickfacts.census.gov/qfd/states/36/36103.html

Chen, L. M., Orav, E. J., & Epstein, A. M. (2012). Public reporting on risk-adjusted mortality after percutaneous coronary interventions in New York State: Forecasting ability and impact on market share and physicians' decisions to discontinue practice. *Circulation: Cardiovascular Quality and Outcomes, 5*(1), 70–75. doi:10.1161/CIRCOUTCOMES.111.962761

Coombs, M. (2003). Power and conflict in intensive care clinical decision making. *Intensive and Critical Care Nursing, 19*(3), 125–135.

Cosby, K. S., & Croskerry, P. (2004). Profiles in patient safety: Authority gradients in medical error. *Academic Emergency Medicine, 11*(12), 1341–1345. doi:10.1197/j.aem.2004.07.005

Donchin, Y., Gopher, D., Olin, M., Badihi, Y., Biesky, M., Sprung, C. L., . . . Cotev, S. (1995). A look into the nature and causes of human errors in the intensive care unit. *Critical Care Medicine, 23*(2), 294–300.

Friedman, M. I., Cooper, A. H., Click, E., & Fitzpatrick, J. J. (2011). Specialized new graduate RN critical care orientation: Retention and financial impact. *Nursing Economics, 29*(1), 7–14.

Hannan, E. L., Cozzens, K., King, S. B., III, Walford, G., & Shah, N. R. (2012). The New York State cardiac registries: History, contributions, limitations, and lessons for future efforts to assess and publicly report healthcare outcomes. *Journal of the American College of Cardiology, 59*(25), 2309–2316. doi:10.1016/j.jacc.2011.12.051

Kohn, L. T., Corrigan, J., & Donaldson, M. S. (2000). *To err is human: Building a safer health system*. Washington, DC: National Academy Press.

Manojlovich, M. (2010). Nurse/physician communication through a sensemaking lens: Shifting the paradigm to improve patient safety. *Medical care, 48*(11), 941–946. doi:10.1097/MLR.0b013e3181eb31bd

Reader, T. W., Flin, R., Mearns, K., & Cuthbertson, B. H. (2007). Interdisciplinary communication in the intensive care unit. *British Journal of Anaesthesia, 98*(3), 347–352. doi:10.1093/bja/ael372

Roth, M. D., & Daze, A. M. (1984). Are nurses practicing medicine in the ICU? *Dimensions of Critical Care Nursing, 3*(4), 230–237.

Salas, E., DiazGranados, D., Weaver, S. J., & King, H. (2008). Does team training work? Principles for health care. *Academic Emergency Medicine, 15*(11), 1002–1009. doi:10.1111/j.1553-2712.2008.00254.x

Shortell, S. M., Zimmerman, J. E., Rousseau, D. M., Gillies, R. R., Wagner, D. P., Draper, E. A., . . . Duffy, J. (1994). The performance of intensive care units: Does good management make a difference? *Medical Care, 32*(5), 508–525.

Smith, M. (1998). Who should run intensive care units? *Care of the Critically Ill, 14*(4), 113–115.

Thomas, E. J., Sexton, J. B., & Helmreich, R. L. (2003). Discrepant attitudes about teamwork among critical care nurses and physicians. *Critical Care Medicine, 31*(3), 956–959. doi:10.1097/01.CCM.0000056183.89175.76

Kristy Loewenstein
James Roth

5: More Than Mock Codes: Simulation for Management of the Medically Ill Patient in a Psychiatric Setting

Behavioral health patients are expected to be cleared and medically stable prior to in-patient admittance. In years past this was always the case, but recent psychiatric admissions include complex patients, often with multiple comorbidities, who may at some time during hospitalization require emergency treatment and transfer. Mental health professionals are frequently not comfortable, confident, or competent in current best practice management of such cases. A simulation program in a psychiatric hospital aims to prevent harm to patients when such incidents occur. Crafted for registered nurses, nurse practitioners, and resident physicians, it fosters teamwork and collaboration while enabling deliberate practice to improve emergency skills in a safe and protected setting.

Mortality rates are higher among patients with serious psychiatric disorders (Harris & Barraclough, 1998) than for the general population. Longevity may be reduced by as much as 30%, with typical life spans that are 15 to 30 years shorter than average, according to one analysis of public mental health records in the United States (Colton & Manderscheid, 2006). Cardiovascular disease is the most common cause of death (Curkendall, Mo, Glasser, Rose Stang, & Jones, 2004), while at highest risk for premature death (both from natural and

TABLE 5.1 Clinical Antipsychotic Trials of Intervention Effectiveness (CATIE)

■ More than 1,400 schizophrenic patients in trial, compared effectiveness of first- and second-generation antipsychotics

■ Trials also collected data that 58% of patients enrolled had at least one medical comorbidity

■ 9 percent of patients had 4 or more medical conditions

■ Hypertension (HTN) was the number one medical co-morbidity in patients enrolled in CATIE; 20% of all patients enrolled had HTN; 14% had hyperlipidemia

Source: Table 1 From Chwastiak et al 2006.

unnatural causes) among patients with serious mental illness are those who suffer from substance abuse, eating disorders, schizophrenia, and depression.

Physicians may frequently underestimate the pretest probability of disease and order fewer appropriate tests for patients with common medical complaints (headache, abdominal pain) and comorbid psychiatric illness (Graber et al., 2000). Many patients report that they postpone care because they do not believe health care staff will believe them (DeCoux, 2005; Goldberg et al., 2007). Suggested approaches to physical assessment are several. Nurses and psychiatrists need to be aware of stigma and their own biases. They should listen carefully, review medical records, and contact collateral sources of information as needed. Most importantly, they should not ignore the patient but operate with a high index of suspicion for medical comorbidity in specific clinical situations—decompensation without a clear stressor or precipitant, for example, especially in the face of compliance to medication. Similarly, a history of "psychiatric" signs or symptoms, such as can occur in patients with developmental disabilities, may mask an underlying medical condition. Health care providers should also be attuned to odd requests for intervention and they need to be wary of too hastily attributing medical complaints to psychiatric symptoms or behaviors. They should consider instead obtaining more objective data (vital signs, labs) and seek consultation when there are barriers to medical evaluation.

Raising Standards for Managing Medical Emergencies

At Zucker Hillside Hospital (ZHH), a 221-bed behavioral health facility on Long Island, New York (part of the North Shore Long Island Jewish [NS-LIJ] Health System), which offers a full range of services including inpatient and ambulatory electroconvulsive therapy, we developed a simulation course with a specially designed curriculum to help nurses and resident psychiatrists manage evolving medical emergencies. Most commonly, we see patients with the most complex and medically unstable problems on two inpatient geriatric units, but adult and adolescent patients may also be admitted with co-occurring medical disorders. Our program, inaugurated in 2010, exposes participants to simulated but challenging scenarios.

Few psychiatric hospitals are equipped to care for seriously medically compromised patients; cardiac arrest and/or death are unexpected outcomes. Increasingly, however, mental health patients with medical comorbidities are admitted to behavioral health facilities where nurses and psychiatrists may not be certified in advanced cardiac life support (ACLS) and do not have sufficient knowledge concerning, or access to, appropriate drugs. At ZHH, where we maintain a basic life support (BLS) standard of care, our medical equipment is limited and we transfer unstable patients to the adjacent tertiary care facility.

About 2005 we began to see an increase in the number of complex patients being admitted to ZHH and recognized that nurses and physicians were not comfortable managing their infrequent but essentially inevitable medical emergencies. In one instance, when a patient suffered cardiac arrest, the attending nurse and physician delayed cardiopulmonary resuscitation (CPR); in another case, staff experienced difficulty managing a patient with a gastrointestinal (GI) bleed. As a consequence, our education departments for both the nursing and residency programs looked toward developing remediation to improve the staff's competence and comfort level in terms of emergency treatment and transfer.

Our initial focus concerned resuscitation certification. Prior to 2007, training in CPR was not standardized. Some nurses had taken the BLS course offered by the American Heart Association (AHA); others were trained in AHA's less rigorous Heartsaver CPR automatic external defibrillator (AED) course; still others had certification from organizations such as the American Red Cross. Nor did all mental health workers (MHWs), except nursing students and transfers from the children's hospital, have documented CPR certification. Consequently, beginning in late 2007, CPR certification became a job requirement for all registered nurses, and in 2009 all MHWs were required to pass the AHA's Heartsaver AED course. By early 2010 all psychiatric assistants were also certified.

Use of Mock Codes

Mock codes with a task trainer manikin represented an additional move toward improved safety. Beginning in late 2007 we initiated code drills and held them four times each month, in hospital and on varying units—two on the day or evening shift, and two during the night shift. An educator/assistant director of nursing brought the CPR manikin to the unit, and all available nursing staff participated. Staff members were required to demonstrate CPR skills, to bring the AED to the "patient" while being monitored for response time to start CPR, and to deploy the apparatus. They were also to know the location of all equipment and how to make the requisite emergency phone calls. We revised this aspect of the program in 2009 to ensure by verbal assessment that staff knew the circumstances in which to use, and how to operate, the various equipment (backboard, suction, O_2, EKG, and pulse oximetry), how to assign a code leader, and how to assess an unresponsive and/or unconscious patient discovered in bed or in a chair. We required ancillary staff to know emergency phone numbers and be able to describe what they would do to locate the emergency cart if they were assigned the beeper and had to respond.

We further enhanced this program by adding instructors, providing additional rapid response information, and requiring compliance verified by attestation. Assistant nurse managers now run 30 mock codes each month, which are monitored as a performance improvement initiative. Our nurse educators enter relevant data into a spreadsheet, including any problems or comments; staff members requiring remediation are directed to nursing education. We also created an interface with the residency program to train staff in teams. Residents now attend monthly mock drills; nursing education helps to orient new residents in a medical skills lab, where we use the simulation phlebotomy arm, the AED simulator, and instruct all new residents concerning the hospital's emergency procedures and equipment. In 2013, we also started a medical skills review class for second- and third-year residents.

In all, CPR certification, mock codes, and new medical equipment represented a reasonable beginning to help resolve the problem of staff confidence and competence in dealing with medical emergencies in a behavioral health setting. But in medicine generally, more than 20 years' experience with training personnel in resuscitation has underscored the limitations of both knowledge and skills retention in this kind of training (Hamilton, 2005). Owing to low rates of success with cardiovascular emergencies, some hospitals have instituted a full-scale redesign of basic and advanced CPR instruction (Lighthall, Mayette, & Hamilton, 2013). In our view, to ensure a positive impact on patient safety and patient outcomes, high-fidelity simulation was an avenue we needed to explore. Our adult learners could benefit from a safe environment that afforded hands-on experiential learning to contend with unexpected life-threatening events. CPR might have value in teaching manual skills and a basic approach to cardiovascular emergencies, but it did not provide sufficient focus on teamwork, communications, or critical thinking to be reliably expected to transfer medical management skills to the clinical setting in real time.

Evolution of a Behavioral Health Medical Emergency Course Using High-Fidelity Simulation

In consultation with the Patient Safety Institute (PSI), we designed a course that uses high-fidelity simulation to address the several interrelated issues noted previously: continued and fairly frequent transfers between our psychiatric hospital and the medical facility, several poor outcomes in clinical emergencies, and the insufficiency of mock codes. Course development followed a stepwise path shaped in part by the paucity of literature specific to medical emergencies in psychiatric hospitals (Puskar, Smith, Hersiko, & Urda, 2011). Initially, we met with the leadership of PSI to outline the aims and to learn the basic parameters of simulation. Subsequently, nurse educators, assistant nurse managers and staff nurses, and the residency program director all took the institute's simulation instructor course, which provided a framework for the program we then developed, consistent with its underlying philosophy and educational methodologies.

We should note at the outset that, for our psychiatric personnel, the consistent use of "debriefing with good judgment" that followed each simulation scenario represented a ready and useful extension of their preexisting skills (see Chapter 2). In general, behavioral clinicians constantly work with verbal information to assess patients and provide care; they are not prone to anxiety in discussing emotionally toned issues and they generally learn how to manage conflict and avoid damaging confrontations with patients and colleagues.[1] In addition, residents and nurses at ZHH are familiar with debriefings in the hospital setting; these take place systematically after episodes of restraint and other similar incidents. As a consequence, it seemed, both instructors and participants rapidly came to understand that the postsimulation debrief was the most important part of the course, where the greatest share of learning takes place. Guided both by the instructor who observed the scenario and a facilitator from PSI, the teams were able to deploy critical thinking and collectively and constructively work to discuss their hands-on management of

---

COURSE OUTLINE

- Prework: Assessment of Medical Problems in Acute Psychiatric Patients and Medical Comorbidity in Mental Health Patients (PowerPoint Presentation)
- Pretest (15 minutes)
- Handout: Medical Emergency Decision Tree (see Figure 5.1)
- Simulations and debriefs (2.5 hours)
- Medical equipment review (45 minutes)
- Posttest, course evaluations, and questions (30 minutes)

Pretest or posttest (please circle)   Class Date:_____

1. You find a patient in bed, with no pulse, and not breathing. What is the correct hospital code to call when you dial "22?"
   a. Medical Emergency
   b. Rapid Response
   c. Psychiatric Emergency
   d. Code Blue

2. The following equipment is not available for use during a medical emergency at ZHH:
   a. Portable suction
   b. AED
   c. Grab and Go O_2
   d. Intubation tray

3. The correct ratio for compressions to breaths in cardiopulmonary resuscitation is:
   a. 5:2
   b. 15:2
   c. 30:2
   d. 15:5

4. What is the correct initial intervention for a choking victim who is found unresponsive?
   a. Heimlich maneuver
   b. Initiate oxygen therapy
   c. Initiate CPR
   d. Suction patient's airway

5. What is the appropriate response to a patient experiencing an active seizure?
   a. Hold the patient down
   b. Place something in the patient's mouth to prevent from biting himself or herself
   c. Turn patient to the side to prevent aspiration
   d. Put side rails up, if applicable, and note how long the seizure lasts

6. You are on the geriatric psychiatry unit at the 7 p.m. RN shift change and go to check on your 85-year-old patient. She is complaining of headache and dizziness and blurred vision with a BP of 160/88. What is the appropriate action to take?
   a. Call the intern on call and stay with the patient
   b. Call the Rapid Response code and discuss with the IOC the need to call NS-LIJ ambulance to transfer the patient
   c. Encourage the patient to drink more fluids and repeat vitals in 20 minutes
   d. Give a Nitrostat tab and check to see if she has relief in 30 minutes

7. You find a patient sitting in a chair, slumped over, in the dayroom. You try to assess for a pulse, and cannot palpate one. The patient is not breathing. You call for help. What is the appropriate action to take next?
   a. Leave the patient to call "22"
   b. Transfer patient to the floor and begin CPR
   c. Try to ventilate the patient while the patient is in the chair
   d. Get a fingerstick

8. A patient has been complaining of abdominal pain for a few days. All vital signs have been within normal limits, but at 8 p.m., prior to medication time, the patient tells you he is vomiting blood, and several minutes later you witness him vomiting dark, coffee ground-colored fluid. What is the appropriate action to take?
   a. Offer the patient TUMS® with his meds
   b. Attempt to suction the patient
   c. Stay with the patient and instruct another staff member to call "Rapid Response" and NS-LIJ ambulance
   d. Call a "Code Blue" and stay with the patient

9. A patient that was choking has become unconscious. The correct sequence of steps to take next is:
   a. Assist patient to the floor, straddle patient, and perform abdominal thrusts
   b. Call for help, assist patient to the floor, and begin CPR
   c. Assist patient to the floor, suction patient, and perform abdominal thrusts
   d. Try to sweep out in the patient's mouth

10. An alcohol-addicted patient has started to experience withdrawal and has begun to seize. The IOC arrives on the unit and tells the nurse he wants to give the patient Ativan via IV. What would be the correct response from the RN?
    a. I am not competencied to start an IVs, but I can prime the line and prepare it for you
    b. What dose of Ativan would you like to give?
    c. I do not know how to start an IV
    d. We don't do IVs here

the patient and their ability to meet the preset goals of the simulation, including use of basic life support equipment and procedures for escalation.

The class, as we developed it for both nurses and resident psychiatrists, is hands-on and practical. Students participate in scenarios involving deteriorating patients, including cardiac arrest. A single session engages all participants in three separate scenarios: "Code Blue" (cardiac/respiratory arrest); "Critical Upper Airway Response" (choking response simulation); and "Alcohol Withdrawal," which includes seizures. We recently added a fourth scenario: "Suicide Attempt." All scenarios utilize high-fidelity manikins that simulate breathing and pulse; they

SCENARIO #1: CODE BLUE

The nurse enters to discover the patient seated in a chair with no pulse and no respiration. The team responds to her call, works together to assess according to AHA guidelines and start BLS, including use of the AED. They use the glucometer to check blood sugar and they apply oxygen (to be used with the ambu-bag). Once the patient is successfully resuscitated, after calling Code Blue and while awaiting emergency medical services (EMS), the team should obtain an electrocardiogram (EKG).

are controlled by a remote "wizard" (director of the scenario) from the control/observation booth who also speaks to the staff as the voice of the patient.

In Scenario #1, a nurse usually enters the room first and finds the patient unconscious. The nurse assesses for responsiveness; there is none. The nurse

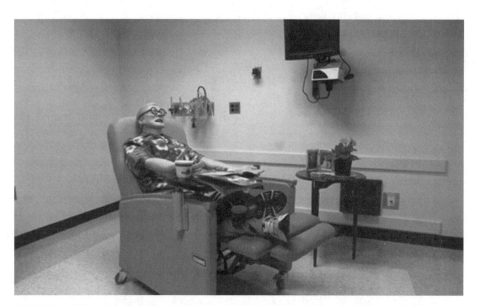

FIGURE 5.1 The high-fidelity simulation manikin positioned in the "day room" at the start of Scenario #1.

calls for help and the other team members, usually three RNs, enter to assist. They must use critical thinking to determine the nature of the situation. Since the patient is discovered in a chair with no pulse and is not breathing, the RN should announce a Code Blue. One of the staff should initiate a telephone call to EMS, which actually reaches a nursing instructor observing the scenario. The team, by prior instruction, should be aware that at ZHH two phone calls are required: an internal call to the page operator, who transmits a Code Blue alert to the pager system; and another call, to NS-LIJ EMS. The second call re-inforces provision of correct, orderly, and vital information that enables transfer of the patient to the health system's emergency department; its accuracy affects decision-making on the part of EMS, which determines who among the staff—normally, an emergency medical technician (EMT) or paramedic—to deploy.

After Code Blue is called, the resident enters. At this point in the scenario, the team should have moved their patient from the chair to the floor to initiate CPR. The three nurses and physician now constitute the team treating the patient and they need to work and communicate together for the scenario to be successful.

Observation of this scenario frequently notes aspects of participants' behavior in both time and space, which we discuss at length during the debrief. To perform CPR in the hospital room setting, the patient must be lifted off the chair and placed on the floor. Frequently, team members fail to assume the right position, backing into a corner or in some way unable to properly perform the head tilt chin lift (for breaths), or to position themselves beside the patient (for compression). That these difficulties regularly occur despite CPR training suggests the role stress can play in unfamiliar situations.

Similarly, when the AED apparatus alerts team members to perform compression for 2 full minutes, they discover that the duration can seem unduly long in a life-threatening simulation. They often behave as though the machine is broken, stopping compression to verify the timing. Preshock chest compression

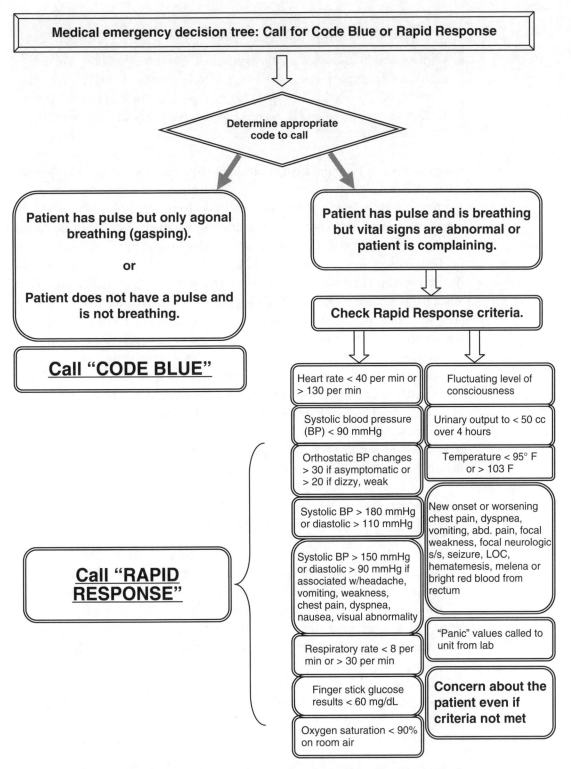

FIGURE 5.2 The Zucker Hillside Hospital Response Criteria Decision Tree for medical
emergencies.

SCENARIO #2 : CRITICAL UPPER AIRWAY OBSTRUCTION

Choking and in distress, the patient arrives at the nursing station, and then darts into the hospital room. The team follows and enters to find the patient on the floor, unconscious. Helping to turn the patient over, the nurse starts CPR. A second staff member attempts suction and applies a pulse oximeter.

---

interruptions can have negative clinical consequences (Souchtchenko, Benner, Allen, & Brady, 2013).

Our second scenario, a variation on Code Blue, starts abruptly. While the team is being prebriefed outside a patient's hospital room, a standardized patient (portrayed by a PSI staff member) appears suddenly, coughing and choking. He or she is dressed in a distinctive shirt identical to the one that the team will find on the manikin. The patient's appearance alerts the team to premorbid signs; then, when they enter the room, they find the patient (manikin) on the floor, unresponsive. With the difference that the patient must be checked for airway obstruction, this scenario now plays out like the first, with the same expected outcomes.

Incidents of dysphagia and choking are relatively common and can present serious, even life-threatening problems for psychiatric in patients (Aldridge & Taylor, 2011). Although choking is often food related, both choking and dysphagia may be due to medication, developmental disorders, or oligodontia and other dental-related issues; some patients will eat too quickly without chewing. Psychiatric nurses and residents have frequently experienced such cases first-hand; so, during the debrief to this scenario, they are often vocal and discuss similar events

---

SCENARIO #3: ALCOHOL WITHDRAWAL SYNDROME

A patient with a known history of alcohol abuse begins to show signs of withdrawal, including elevated blood pressure and rapid pulse, vomiting, seizures, and hallucinations (see Figure 5.3). The medical team will assess vital signs, perform a specific assessment with a validated tool, and administer medication (McKay, Koranda, & Axen, 2004; Sullivan, Sykora, Schneiderman, Naranjo, & Sellers, 1989). They will take precautions with seizures, including timing their duration, documenting whether the patient is incontinent, and noting any response to medication. The physician will decide to have the patient transferred to the emergency department and start an IV prior to transport.

---

encountered in the clinical setting. In the safe environment at PSI, their contributions help develop trust and a sense of security among team members.

Assessment through extensive interrogation makes the third scenario in our series quite different from the first two. The team enters the room to find the

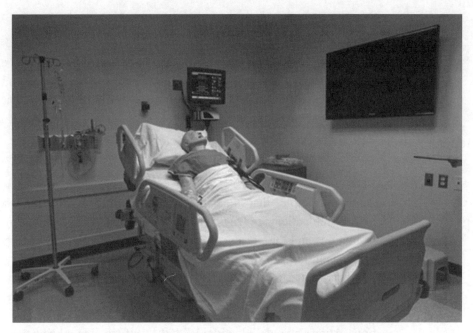

FIGURE 5.3 High-fidelity manikin staged for the alcohol withdrawal scenario.

patient—a manikin—in bed, verbal and alert, but confused. He starts speaking to the nurse but his speech is somewhat garbled, and he grows agitated and belligerent. After several minutes, the patient vomits. (The high-fidelity manikin does not have the capability to simulate vomitus; we use a computerized sound effect.) The staff is expected to put on gloves, provide an emesis basin, and ensure the patient does not aspirate. Soon after vomiting, the patient starts to seize. (The manikin does simulate convulsions.[2]) Included in the mock chart that we prepare for this simulation is a scale to quantify the risk for alcohol withdrawal syndrome, which can lead to serious and sometimes fatal outcomes[3] (McKay, Koranda, & Axen, 2004; Sullivan et al., 1989). The patient seizes several times during the scenario; the nurses are expected to time the seizures and provide that information to the physician. The nurse should call Rapid Response and make another call to request the health service ambulance, providing pertinent information, including the number and duration of seizures, the Clinical Institute Withdrawal Assessment (CIWA) score, and other vital signs. (We use the SBAR [Situation, Background, Assessment, and Recommendation] format from Team-STEPPS®; Fay-Hillier, Regan, & Gallagher Gordon, 2012). The remote physician may request IV administration of lorazepam, a benzodiazepine. Although nurses at ZHH are not trained to start IVs, they can prime the IV line and prepare it for the resident; often, the resident will choose instead to have the nurse administer the medication intramuscularly.

Debriefs for this scenario tend to be wide ranging and rich in content, both because they are frequent occurrences in practice and involve both psychiatric and medical skills. They help clarify roles and responsibilities and review aspects of specific hospital protocol, such as our rule concerning proper positioning of the patient when vomiting. They also offer an opportunity to clarify more

---

SCENARIO #4: SUICIDE ATTEMPT

A nurse discovers a patient who has just slashed his wrist. The smuggled knife he used is partly visible when the nurse enters the room to find him in bed, with extensive and continuing arterial blood loss. The patient is alert but confused, and if immediate action is not taken he will show signs of hypovolemic shock, followed by cardiac arrest.

---

general principles that underscore the difficulties in properly assessing behavioral health patients in ways that can distinguish specific pathological symptom formations and the presence of underlying medical conditions requiring emergency attention.

This scenario, inspired by a recent article (Lilly, Hermanns, & Crawley, 2012), is a combination medical and psychiatric emergency. When the nurse finds the patient in bed, he is awake and talking; his extemporaneous verbalizations express suicidal ideation. With the knife visible in the patient's waistband, we expect the nurse to immediately call for help but also remain cognizant of his or her own personal safety by carefully retrieving the weapon. The rest of the team enters to assess the patient for further injuries and to stabilize bleeding with a pressure dressing or tourniquet while awaiting transfer via EMS.

Debriefs for this scenario include both the psychiatric and medical issues surrounding suicide attempts. The latter include assessing the relative severity of blood loss in a wrist-cutting episode with the attendant risk of arrhythmia, hypovolemic shock, and, if untreated, cardiac arrest and death. Personal safety is also a crucial part of this scenario and an important issue to underscore in behavioral health nursing practice.

Developing Preliminary Data and Future Directions

On an empirical basis we have not experienced poor outcomes for patients as a result of staff members' lack of knowledge or competence in organizing and administrating rapid responses in the clinical setting. In general, we have long held post-hoc discussions with staff and patients after each psychiatric emergency or episode of restraint; we currently also conduct debriefs with the staff in real time after instances of Rapid Response and Code Blue. This allows us to assess the situation, analyze the effectiveness of our patient care, and identify any areas that need immediate remediation. For staff, debriefs can also enhance confidence and ensure closure after an event, providing positive feedback for competent and effective performance.

In general, the rapid response team (RRT) model is widely used in U.S. hospitals and has been extensively implemented in non-ICU settings (Leach, Mayo, & O'Rourke, 2010). The basic reason is straightforward. In such circumstances, "Delays in providing needed care to hospitalized patients whose conditions are deteriorating may increase the likelihood of cardiac arrest or death . . ." (Williams,

Newman, Jones, & Woodard, 2011). Systematic reviews of these protocols come to varying conclusions but they have yet to include behavioral health sites; our search of the literature was null as concerned RRTs, rapid response systems (RRS), or medical emergency teams (METs) in inpatient psychiatry, mental health, or behavioral health settings. At ZHH we adapted our decision tree (see Figure 5.1) from our medical center as a corrective action several years ago in the wake of a poor patient outcome; we subsequently noted an increase in transfers and admissions to the medical center.

As one consequence and in alignment with our resort to simulation, we have started to study the underlying rationale and procedures associated with medical transfers owing to emergencies in a psychiatric facility. In 2012, as part of a performance improvement initiative, the nursing department at ZHH began to attend to and monitor every instance of rapid response in order to collect data on the type of call, the reason for the call, and basic information about the patient, including the number and kind of preexisting comorbidities. We then applied for institutional review board approval for a study, "Behavioral Health Nurses and the Initiation and Sequelae of Rapid Response Team Calls," a retrospective chart review of 100 rapid response team calls attended by nursing administration. The rationale for conducting this study is to add to the body of literature concerning RRTs, and to analyze their use and benefit, if any, for inpatient behavioral health hospitals. Based on findings after the phase of data analysis is complete, we may institute changes to the scenarios in our simulation classes.

NOTES

1. Every staff member is also trained in the TeamSTEPPS® approach, which helps facilitate closed-loop communication.
2. In general, the seizure function with high-fidelity manikins, which can be triggered remotely, may appear more consistent with shivering than with genuine convulsions. For that reason, PSI also uses a mattress with an electropneumatic plate. Note that while, in principle, a standardized patient could be used with this scenario in place of a manikin, actors portraying seizures could pose a safety risk to themselves.
3. We use the revised Clinical Institute Withdrawal Assessment (CIWA-AR), a widely researched and reliable instrument.

REFERENCES

Aldridge, K., & Taylor, N. F. (2012). Dysphagia is a common and serious problem for adults with mental illness: A systematic review. *Dysphagia, 27*(1), 124–137. Retrieved from http://www .ncbi.nlm.nih.gov/pubmed/22120763

Chwastiak, L. A., Rosenheck, R. A., McEvoy, J. P., Keefe, R. S., Swartz, M. S., & Lieberman, J. A. (2006). Interrelationships of psychiatric symptom severity, medical comorbidity, and functioning in schizophrenia. *Psychiatric Services, 57*(8), 1102–1109. doi:10.1176/appi.ps.57.8.1102

Colton, C., & Manderscheid, R. (2006). Congruencies in increased mortality rates, years of potential life lost, and causes of death among public mental health clients in eight states. *Preventing Chronic Disease, 3*(2), A42.

Curkendall, S., Mo, J., Glasser, D. B., Rose Stang, M., & Jones, J. (2004). Cardiovascular disease in patients with schizophrenia in Saskatchewan, Canada. *Journal of Clinical Psychiatry, 65*(5), 715–720.

Decoux M. (2005). Acute versus primary care: The health care decision making process for individuals with severe mental illness. *Issues in Mental Health Nursing, 26*(9), 935–951.

Fay-Hillier, T., Regan, R. V., & Gallagher Gordon, M. (2012). Communication and patient safety in simulation for mental health nursing education. *Issues in Mental Health Nursing.* Retrieved from http://www.ncbi.nlm.nih.gov/pubmed/23146005

Goldberg, R., Kreyenbuhl, J., Medoff, D., Dickerson, F., Wohlheiter, K., Fang, L. J., . . . Dixon, L. B. (2007). Quality of diabetes care among adults with serious mental illness. *Psychiatric Services, 58*(4), 536–543.

Graber, M., Bergus, G., Dawson, J. D., Wood, G. B., Levy, B. T., & Levin, I. (2000). Effect of a patient's psychiatric history on physicians' estimation of probability of disease. *Journal of General Internal Medicine, 15*(3), 204–206.

Hamilton, R. (2005). Nurses' knowledge and skill retention following cardiopulmonary resuscitation training: A review of the literature. *Journal of Advanced Nursing.* Retrieved from http://www.ncbi.nlm.nih.gov/pubmed/16033596

Harris, E. & Barraclough, B. (1998). Excess mortality of mental disorder. *British Journal of Psychiatry, 173,* 11–53.

Leach, L., Mayo, A., & O'Rourke, M. (2010). "How RNs rescue patients: A qualitative study of RN's perceived involvement in rapid response teams." *Quality and Safety in Health Care, 19,* e13.

Lighthall, G., Mayette, M., & Hamilton, T. K. (2013). An institutionwide approach to redesigning management of cardiopulmonary resuscitation. *The Joint Commission Journal on Quality and Patient Safety.* Retrieved from http://www.ncbi.nlm.nih.gov/pubmed/23641535

Lilly, M., Hermanns, & M., Crawley, B. (2012). Psychiatric nursing emergency: A simulated experience of a wrist-cutting suicide attempt. *Journal of Psychosocial Nursing, 50*(2), 35–42.

McKay, A., Koranda, A., & Axen, D. (2004). Using a symptomtriggered approach to manage patients in acute alcohol withdrawal. *Medsurg Nursing.* Retrieved from http://www.ncbi.nlm.nih.gov/pubmed/15029927

NIMH Clinical Antipsychotic Trials of Intervention Effectiveness CATIE. www.nimh.nih.gov. Retrieved from http://www.nimh.nih.gov/funding/clinical-trials-for-researchers/practical/catie/index.shtml. Accessed june 30, 2014.

Puskar, K., Smith, M. D., Hersiko, C., & Urda, B. (2011). Medical emergencies in psychiatric hospitals. *Issues in Mental Health Nursing.* Retrieved from http://www.ncbi.nlm.nih.gov/pubmed/?term=puskar+medical+emergencies+2011.

Souchtchenko, S., Benner, J. P., Allen, J. L., & Brady, W. J. (2013). A review of chest compression interruptions during out-of-hospital cardiac arrest and strategies for the future. *Journal Emergency Medicine.* Retrieved from http://dx.doi.org/10.1016/j.jemermed.2013.01.023. Accessed June 30, 2014.

Sullivan, J., Sykora, K., Schneiderman, J., Naranjo, CA., & Sellers, EM. (1989). Assessment of alcohol withdrawal the revised clinical institute withdrawal assessment for alcohol scale (CIWA-Ar). *British Journal of Addiction.* Retrieved from http://www.ncbi.nlm.nih.gov/pubmed/2597811.

Williams, D., Newman, A., Jones, C., & Woodard, B. (2011). "Nurses' perceptions of how rapid response teams affect the nurse, team and system." *Journal of Nursing Care Quality, 26*(3), 265–272.

Michael Cassara
Robert L. Kerner Jr.
Andrew Drozd

6: Creating High-Fidelity and Hybrid Simulations for Residents in Emergency Medicine

An accredited 3-year training program for emergency medicine (EM) residents at a tertiary care hospital employed simulation-based education (SBE), initially for limited educational objectives and assessment purposes. The program expanded with advances in high-fidelity capabilities and expert faculty but remained on a limited schedule before embarking upon collaboration with the health system's corporate university and dedicated simulation center. This chapter details the program's development over time together with current theory and practice in crafting scenarios that both augment the accepted model curriculum and integrate it to meet the needs of millennial residents.

Simulation plays an integral role in the education and assessment of today's EM residents. Its use as a primary andragogy within EM training programs has grown exponentially over the past 3 decades (McLaughlin, Bond, Promes & Spillane, 2006; Okuda et al., 2008). Reasons for the expanded integration of simulation within these programs include rapid advances in, and greater availability of, simulation technologies; the maturation of increasing numbers of faculty with expertise in applying them; the progressive realization that SBE for adult millennial medical learners appears more effective than other strategies for their assimilation of knowledge, skills, and attitudes required for safe patient care and multidisciplinary, interprofessional collaborative practice; and, finally, the need to fulfill the mandate of external stakeholders for more robust learner assessments. As substantial investments

in infrastructure and faculty development have become commonplace in EM
residency programs, so have evolved the complexity, fidelity, and sophistication
of instructional design. This chapter discusses the background and basic theory
of SBE for today's EM residents, followed by a description of the accredited
program used to teach them in the North Shore-LIJ Health System (NS-LIJ)
together with some of the specific methods used to create simulation-based
experiences.

BACKGROUND AND THEORETICAL BASIS

EM is the specialty dedicated to the diagnosis and treatment of unforeseen illness or injury (American College of Emergency Physicians [ACEP], 2008). It
focuses on the initial assessment, stabilization, management, and disposition
of one or more acutely ill or injured adult or pediatric patients with medical,
traumatic, surgical, obstetrical, or psychiatric conditions. EM is most commonly
practiced in a hospital-based or freestanding emergency department, an urgent
care clinic, an emergency medical response vehicle, or at a disaster site (ACEP,
2008). Inherently complex, EM in practice is variously described as "chaotic,"
"unpredictable," "dynamic," and "fast-paced." The reason for such complexity
and variability lies with its core altruistic mission: to provide care for any patient
with any problem at any time, often with little to no background information,
without the familiarity and insight normally available as part of an established
physician–patient relationship, and without regard for the patient's ability to pay.

Since its recognition as the 23rd medical specialty in the United States
in 1979 (American Board of Emergency Medicine [ABEM], 2013), EM has
become one of the most popular specialties. Competition among medical students for positions in residency programs is extremely high in the United States
because completion of an accredited program is the only available route to certification. Today, there are currently over 170 EM residencies throughout the
United States (Society for Academic Emergency Medicine, 2014). These programs are 3 or 4 years in duration and, upon completion, graduates enter the
workforce as independent practitioners with eligibility for board certification by
the ABEM or the American Osteopathic Board of Emergency Medicine. Graduates may also elect to obtain further subspecialty training in medical toxicology,
pediatric EM, emergency medical services, undersea and hyperbaric medicine,
sports medicine, critical care medicine, or hospice and palliative care. Society
expects that emergency physicians, as professionals completing the prescribed
training pathway for certification, will provide efficient, high-quality, patient-
centered, evidence-based, cost-effective care that is safe and without increased
risk for causing iatrogenic harm. In today's health care environments, this
means that emergency physicians must be able to rapidly access, retrieve, and
apply previously learned knowledge and skills. They also must be able to evaluate and assimilate new information, proficiencies, and perspectives, and they
must collaborate, communicate, and work with the other members of a multidisciplinary, interprofessional team. In addition, they must be at their best when

the circumstances are most challenging, when patient acuity is highest, when temporal influences are greatest, and when the potential consequences are most critical. The primary goal of EM residency programs is to prepare EM residents so they meet these societal expectations.

How to best train emergency physicians for the complicated work they do has been the subject of much deliberation in recent decades and come under increasing scrutiny and debate. Part of the reason for this owes to the way training was conducted in the early history of EM and its inherent risks. Residency programs trained learners primarily using what may be described as a "situated learning (or experiential) model" that was supplemented with weekly in-classroom, lecture-based didactics. Most learning occurred through direct patient care–centered experiences. Over the 3- to 4-year training period, residents were repeatedly partnered with expert clinicians in quasi "master–apprentice" relationships in the actual environment (e.g., emergency department) where patient care was provided. Learning was believed to occur through "osmosis," by repeatedly embedding residents in the immediate community of emergency physicians and more senior residents in practice. Junior (novice) residents began as "legitimate peripheral participants" (Lave & Wenger, 1991). As less experienced emergency practitioners, they observed more expert emergency clinicians managing actual patients; with time and experience, they were given progressively greater responsibilities and more independence for diagnostic and therapeutic management decisions associated with direct patient care. In the early history of emergency physician training, this graduated autonomy occurred very rapidly and often without direct oversight and supervision ("trial by fire"). Internal or external measures of resident performance were used to indicate competency; residents became "comfortable" managing multiple patients or performing common procedures, for example, and faculty granted "privileges" that allowed the resident more independent practice. One sign of "confirmed" proficiency occurred when more senior residents were allowed to serve as experts ("masters") for newer, more junior residents ("apprentices") In medicine generally, this practice is encapsulated in the mantra "See one, do one, teach one," a classic dogma for generations of physicians-in-training among all specialties.

Although widely disseminated and practiced throughout medicine, medical educators today acknowledge that this paradigm, to "practice" practicing medicine, often without direct oversight by credentialed experts, is ethically unjustifiable. Most medical educators would also agree that the paradigm was often inefficient and ineffective. "See one, do one, teach one" requires the serendipitous presence of clinical material (a patient) with the requisite pathology (an indication) supporting the knowledge or technical/nontechnical skills that the learner (an EM resident) needs to learn. Residents hoping to "practice" managing a specific condition, demonstrate a particular skill, or perform a technique must wait for the teaching moment when a patient in need of such treatment arrives. In addition, the "See one, do one, teach one" model espouses the erroneous assumption that it is merely "practice" (repeated attempts) that "makes perfect." Contrary to this notion, most medical educators today subscribe to the contemporary paradigm, deliberate practice, as key to the development of competence, expertise, and mastery-level performance.

As described by Ericsson (2009) and others, deliberate practice is frequent, continuous, expert-facilitated repetition for the purpose of achieving clinical and technical/nontechnical skill competence, expertise, and mastery. In essence, its mantra is "perfect practice makes perfect" and it has emerged as the preferred training paradigm for medical specialties like EM, which requires sound teamwork, collaboration, communication, and situational awareness coupled with effective decision making, skills application, and complex tasks performed in high-pressure contexts. Deliberate practice is consistent with many aspects of contemporary adult learning theory as described by Knowles (1973, 1980), Kolb (1984), and others (Kolb & Kolb, 2005).

EM residents today may be described as adult millennial medical learners. Their learning focuses around specific goals; they are self-motivated, self-directed learners; they are motivated by the desire to change their role in the "society" ("community of practice") in which they operate; they want to be seen by others as "experts," and must progress from incompetency through competency to mastery to do so. They value multiple opportunities to observe, conceptualize, perform, and actively experiment with content to effectively "learn" (i.e., assimilate into practice). Thus, the deliberate practice model nicely accommodates their needs as learners.

Finally, deliberate practice is consistent with contemporary theory concerning technical skills acquisition among physicians as described by Peyton (1998) and others (Aggarwal, Grantcharov, & Darzi, 2007; Lake & Hamdorf, 2004). This theory holds that adult learners need to possess relevant prerequisite knowledge for performance before skills can be practiced; that, in addition, technical skills need to be deconstructed into component steps before they can be learned; and, finally, that novice operators of technical skills need multiple expert-guided repetitions in the laboratory in order to move through several stages of performance (from unconscious incompetence, to conscious incompetence, to conscious competence, to unconscious competence) before true proficiency and mastery are possible.

The unique body of information that defines and distinguishes the emergency physician is described in the Model of the Clinical Practice of Emergency Medicine ("EM Model"; Perina et al., 2012). First published in 2001 and revised biennially ever since, the EM Model explicitly codifies the breadth, depth, and scope of knowledge and technical/nontechnical skills that all emergency physicians must possess to practice independently. It is a "three-dimensional description of EM clinical practice," in which "three intimately interrelated dimensions—patient acuity, physician tasks, and the listing of conditions and components—together represent the sum" of the variables encountered, influences perceived, and actions taken by emergency physicians when providing patient care (Perina et al., 2012). This document serves as the foundation upon which all EM residency program curricula are based.

Most contemporary medical educators in EM residencies are using SBE with increasingly greater frequency to integrate the principles of deliberate practice and facilitate learning the content as outlined in the EM Model. SBE in most programs includes using one or more of the following techniques, either in isolation or combined as mixed-methodology or hybrid experience (McLaughlin et al., 2006; Noeller et al., 2008; Okuda et al., 2008): hypothetical "what if" questions during case-based oral presentations; low-technology oral certification examination-style simulations; partial task training and procedural skill-associated simulations using synthetic and organic (e.g., biologic, cadaveric) substrates; simulated single- and multiple-patient encounters using computer-based and virtual reality enhanced platforms; simulated patients using standardized, trained actors; and simulated computer manikin simulations of single- and multi-patient encounters.

Using one or more of these SBE techniques within a well-organized and designed curriculum incorporating educators with training in debriefing and feedback offers several advantages. SBE allows control of the timing and sequence of tasks (steps) presented to learners. Removed from the real-world pressures associated with direct patient care in the clinical environment, medical educators have the time to ensure that the learner's knowledge, skills, competence, and attitude are appropriate before attempting care with actual patients. They have the freedom to guide learners at individualized speeds and levels of complexity. SBE also prevents learners from assimilating dangerous behaviors or committing dangerous actions with actual patients, which ultimately reduces costs, such as liability, associated with training. SBE reduces learner anxiety and avoids the potential for iatrogenic harm; learners hone skills in a private, secured environment, protected from medico-legal risk and beyond the scrutiny of coworkers, patients, and other observers. In the simulated environment, learners are free to generate, explore, and test their own hypotheses related to the content they are learning, such as alternative approaches to case management, for example, technical skill performance with nondominant handedness, or different communication techniques on how to deliver bad news. A growing body of evidence demonstrating the safety and efficacy of learner-centric SBE supports the decisions of program directors and educators to develop and maintain robust simulation-based curricula in EM residency programs.

EVOLUTION AND COLLABORATION WITH THE PATIENT SAFETY INSTITUTE

The Emergency Medicine Residency Program (EMRP) at North Shore University Hospital was inaugurated on July 1, 1995 with an entering class of eight residents. It is a 3-year (36-month) program fully accredited by the Accreditation Council for Graduate Medical Education (ACGME). Since its inception, it has grown in size to its current complement of 30 residents (10 per class) and has graduated more than 130 emergency physicians. The EMRP is administered and supported by a program director; there are one or more associate/assistant program directors, a program coordinator, core faculty (medical educators), and other practitioners, administrators, and ancillary and support staff.

Simulation has been one of the andragogies used by core EMRP faculty from the beginning. At first it was used predominantly for educational purposes and formative assessments of residents in focused domains. Examples include oral certification examination-style simulations and partial task training for low-frequency, high-acuity technical skills, such as cricothyrotomy, using biologic substrates (deer heads).

The first of two landmark events in the evolution of the EMRP was acquisition, through a grant in 2002, of SimMan® the department's first computer-enhanced manikin simulator.[1] On-site availability of this technology made possible higher-fidelity SBE. Faculty champions for simulation were identified, resources allocated, and a simulation-based curriculum was drafted. We elected to use the EM Model as the source for most of the curricular content, with an emphasis on resident education in geriatrics, as required by the grant award.

At the outset, a number of factors influenced and delimited implementation of the program. The computer-enhanced manikin simulator required wired connections for the display monitor, computer, air compressor, and power supply. Space was limited to a small conference room or real "unused" patient care areas. Perhaps most importantly, faculty had yet to acquire expertise. The original program was modest in its scope: a series of cases, formulated by faculty, played out with teams of learners (up to five residents) with audiences of as many as 20 residents who attempted to learn vicariously by directly observing the simulation-based exercise. Debriefing took place following these sessions but without effort to understand the learner-specific "frames" (mental representations of the events being simulated) or any rigorous and critical evaluation of the performance. Faculty were required to facilitate all aspects of the sessions, including set-up, moulage, and breakdown of the manikin and the environment; they conducted the case-specific prebriefing, operation ("wizardry") of the computer-enhanced manikin simulator, and the debriefing.

For the NS-LIJ EMRP, as for EM residency programs nationwide, manikin availability was a significant impediment to integration of SBE into the existing curriculum. In 2002, only about one in three programs had access to or used computer-enhanced manikin simulators. Of those with such access, only half used them more than once per year (McLaughlin et al., 2006). Together with inadequate infrastructure, an insufficient number of faculty trained in SBE was a common reason for this less-than-optimal integration. Our experience was the same. We had too few core faculty familiar with the technology, curricular design, emerging principles of SBE, or with best practices for educating adult millennial medical learners. When simulation sessions did occur, significant violations in fidelity and breaks in suspension of disbelief occurred regularly. Efficacy, at first, was obviously limited. Nevertheless, EM residents' interest in and satisfaction with this new learning strategy were surprisingly high. In addition, core faculty who were cognizant of the dynamic health care climate realized that there were several reasons to persevere with implementation. Changes in front-line practice and quality evaluation, such as externally mandated and time-sensitive metrics, started to make clinical bedside teaching increasingly and exceedingly difficult. Continuous incorporation of novel diagnostic and therapeutic technologies (e.g., focused bedside ultrasonography and fiberoptic laryngoscopy), into mainstream EM practice required that all team members (not just residents) recevied regular opportunities for deliberate practice to acquire and maintain competency. Perhaps the largest driver for SBE was the "patient safety crisis" in health care signaled by publication of the Institute of Medicine's report *To Err Is Human* (Kohn et al, 2000) and widespread recognition that to reduce the frequency and consequences of medical errors required more effective, enhanced team training.

Stakeholders within the Department of Emergency Medicine concluded that SBE was not just a transient fad and they made strategic investments to support and foster expansion of the program, both to enable core faculty to obtain the training necessary for simulation-based andragogies and to provide infrastructure, including conversion of revenue-generating patient care space into a one-room simulation laboratory. Within 3 years, a small group of faculty emerged with an enhanced understanding of curricular design and greater knowledge of, and experience with, simulation.

SBE remained scheduled on a quarterly basis, however, until the second landmark event in the evolution of the EMRP: establishment of the Patient Safety Institute (PSI) in 2005. Operating under the aegis of the Center for Learning and Innovation (see Chapter 2), and several times expanded, PSI, together with opening of the Clinical Skills Center in 2011 and reorganization of the BioSkills Center in 2012, had considerable impact on the EMRP. PSI provided access to the latest generation of computer-enhanced manikin simulators, high-technology/high-fidelity partial task trainers, and digital audiovisual recording with playback capability. Faculty development courses included debrief-specific training, simulation "grand rounds," and invited presentations. Further support came from the ability to use standardized patients, the benefit of interprofessional and multidisciplinary expertise, and other logistical, financial, and technical help. We now had opportunities for networking and collaboration, and for sharing experience, research, and scholarship. Because the partnership between the EMRP simulation faculty and administration and PSI was especially strong from the start, the scope and vision of the program expanded rapidly.

From 2006, when we transferred the locus of activity from the hospital to the institute, until the present, the robust proliferation of curricula is a measure of success of the EMRP-PSI collaboration. SBE sessions within the program itself increased in frequency, from quarterly to monthly to weekly, and the simulation faculty grew in number from two in 2002 to more than 25 in 2013. In addition, joint interprofessional, multidisciplinary SBE sessions include nurse fellowship programs in EM and other residency programs throughout the health system; partners include the EM residency program at Long Island Jewish Medical

Center, the medical toxicology fellowship program at North Shore University Hospital (NSUH), a sports medicine fellowship, and the emergency ultrasound fellowship program. Both PSI and the BioSkills Center include EM simulation faculty; so, too, does the newly established Hofstra NS-LIJ School of Medicine.

CURRENT CONCEPTUAL FRAMEWORK

The overall goals of our program today are twofold: to improve the safety and quality of care that EM residents deliver as they progress through the training program; and, with regard to educational outcomes, to produce, upon completion of the residency training program, fully accredited practitioners. To achieve these goals, we incorporate a variety of simulation-based modalities and techniques to enhance each resident's assimilation of higher cognitive, psychomotor, and affective skills. (Table 6.1 provides breakdown usage by modality; Table 6.2 provides a brief overview of some of the content in our SBE program.) The great majority of SBE experiences we provide are high-fidelity, high-technology simulations of single-patient encounters with manikin simulators; but these are not the only modalities we use. We use other strategies in lieu of, or in combination with, high-fidelity simulation as part of hybrid or mixed experiences when specific educational goals and objectives need to be met.

High-fidelity and high-technology simulations have the advantage of incorporating a wide variety of options resembling reality. They "allow [residents] to reason through a clinical problem with little or no cueing, permit [residents] to make life-threatening errors without hurting a real patient, provide instant feedback so [residents] can correct a mistaken action, and rate [residents'] performance on clinical problems that are difficult or impossible to evaluate effectively in other circumstances" (Accreditation Council for Graduate Medical Education [ACGME] & American Board of Medical Specialties [ABMS], 2000). High-fidelity simulations can repeatedly reproduce a variety of standardized scenarios and provide faculty with the opportunity to assess resident performance across multiple domains (e.g., information gathering, patient management, communication skills) during a single educational experience (Swing, 2002). Previous and ongoing research supports the validity and reliability of

TABLE 6.1 Breakdown of SBE Experiences Offered, by Modality

FORMAT	APPROXIMATE PERCENTAGE OF OVERALL SBE EXPERIENCES OFFERED (ANNUALLY)
Computer-enhanced manikin simulator	80%
Task training (cadaver, other biologic,and synthetic substrates)	14%
Oral examination-style (low technology simulation)	5%
Virtual	1%

TABLE 6.2 Brief Summary of Examples of SBE Used in the North Shore University Hospital Simulation Program for Emergency Medicine Residents

SIMULATION-BASED EDUCATIONAL STRATEGY	SIMULATOR	EXAMPLES
Partial task training	Biologic substrates ■ chicken legs ■ harvested deer heads ■ eggs ■ cadavers Synthetic models ■ plastic low-technology manikins (adult, toddler, infant-sized)	■ Intraosseous needle insertion ■ Deer trachea (cricothyrotomy) ■ Slit lamp exam, impression tonometry ■ Endotracheal intubation ■ Video-assisted laryngoscopy ■ Needle/tube thoracostomy ■ Pericardiocentesis ■ Arthrocentesis ■ Thoracotomy
Low-technology simulations	Synthetic models ■ plastic low-technology manikins (adult, toddler, infant-sized)	■ Cardiopulmonary resuscitation training ■ Basic life support technical skill training ■ Advanced cardiac life support case-based simulations ■ Pediatric advanced life support case-based simulations ■ Basic and advanced airway management technical skill training
Role-plays	Verbal simulations ■ case-based scenarios ■ vignettes	■ Simulated oral certification examination-style simulations ■ Hypothetical: "what if" scenarios/explorations during case presentations (during didactic conferences)
High-technology simulations	■ Computer-enhanced manikin simulators (all age ranges: neonatal to geriatric) ■ Sometimes incorporated with partial task trainers to form hybrid simulations ■ Sometimes incorporated with standardized patients to form virtual emergency department ("Sim ED")	■ Complex resuscitations of patients with emergent/critical medical, nontraumatic surgical, traumatic, neurosurgical, toxic-metabolic, and obstetrical/gynecologic emergencies

(continued)

TABLE 6.2 Brief Summary of Examples of SBE Used in the North Shore University Hospital Simulation Program for Emergency Medicine Residents *(continued)*

SIMULATION-BASED EDUCATIONAL STRATEGY	SIMULATOR	EXAMPLES
Standardized patients	n/a	■ Medical resuscitations: agitated patients with toxic-metabolic/psychiatric etiologies; acute stroke ■ Interpersonal and communication skills: breaking bad news, initial baseline Accreditation Council for Graduate Medical Education (ACGME) competency measurement; ongoing milestone assessment
Virtual simulations	■ Proprietary case-based scenarios and vignettes (American Heart Association)	■ Advanced cardiac life support ■ Pediatric advanced life support ■ Basic life support

their use, their effectiveness in teaching procedural and clinical medicine, and their role overall in EM graduate education (McLaughlin et al., 2008 Noeller et al., 2008; Wang et al., 2008).

For effective learning to occur using high-fidelity high-technology simulation, several essential features must be present. We integrate as many evidence-based best practices as possible when designing our curriculum to ensure that the optimal conditions supporting effective learning are present. We use this same approach when designing individual simulation cases. In the sections that follow, we describe these best practices and the evidence basis for them.

FIDELITY AND FEEDBACK: MAJOR CONSIDERATIONS

The single most important component of an effective simulation-based curriculum is feedback. The term "feedback" has three meanings in simulation. According to van de Ridder, Stokking, McGaghie, and ten Cate (2008), one definition of feedback is "information" provided during a simulation to a participant. Feedback is also a "reaction," the modification, consequences, cueing, or effects experienced by a participant during simulation resulting from actions previously taken or decisions previously made. Finally, feedback is a "cycle," the flow of information between learner and instructor. This is perhaps the most commonly applied understanding of feedback; it is operationally defined by van de Ridder et al. (2008) as "specific information about the comparison between a trainee's observed performance and a standard, given with the intent to improve the trainee's performance." Feedback may be built into the simulator, given by the instructor in real time, or provided post hoc in the form of debriefing, a specific type of structured feedback. Debriefing has been demonstrated to be the most essential form of feedback provided to learners during an SBE experience (Issenberg, McGaghie, Petrusa, Lee Gordon, & Scalese, 2005), and there are several styles and formats used, depending on goals and objectives.

To better appreciate the importance of feedback to simulation, consider the distinctions proposed in the preceding. Under the first two meanings, feedback is necessary for learners to maintain their "suspension of disbelief" throughout a simulation experience. Integrity and overall fidelity of the simulation are heightened when the simulation or simulator provide direct case-related feedback to participants that aligns with actions they perform. Failure of the patient's lungs to inflate together with lack of improvement in the pulse oximeter reading that accompanies esophageal intubation represent examples of essential feedback that learners must have and simulation must provide. This "case-in-play" feedback differs from that which faculty provide as part of formative assessment which aims to inform and guide professional growth and development. SBE without debriefing does not result in meaningful learning nor does it create enduring changes in behavior (Issenberg et al., 2005; Motola, Devine, Chung, Sullivan, & Issenberg, 2013). The duration and timing of debriefing have been shown to have important influences upon the learning that results from SBE; quality and impact are best if it takes place immediately following the simulation (Cantrell, 2008; Fanning & Gaba, 2007) and if it allows sufficient time for exploration, analysis, reflection, and discussion of the performances observed (van de Ridder et al., 2008; Van Heukelom, Begaz, & Treat, 2010).

PERCEPTION FIDELITY

Another essential feature we expect of our SBE is fidelity. Khan, Tolhurst-Cleaver, White, and Simpson (2011) describe fidelity as "how realistic the simulation feels, with the emphasis on the 'feelings' or 'perceptions' [of the participant]." Perception fidelity of simulation results from the cumulative influence of several other forms of fidelity:

■ *Mechanical or equipment fidelity* represents "the ability of models or manikins to reproduce the static or dynamic processes on which the simulation is based" (Khan et al., 2011) and refers specifically to the simulator. The term should refer to a specific attribute; it may be misleading if applied to the capabilities of the entire manikin. For example, "a simulator generally regarded as having 'high [mechanical] fidelity' with regard to its respiratory functions may be considered as having low mechanical fidelity if the scenario required the simulator to spontaneously sit up in bed" (Khan et al., 2011). Mechanical fidelity is a major contributor to the perception fidelity of a scenario

■ *Action fidelity* refers to the reproducibility of tasks that participants must perform during a simulation and may involve either technical skills (e.g., thoracostomy tube insertion) or nontechnical skills (e.g., communication with a consultant; Khan et al., 2011). Threats to action fidelity are common and may be related to either the simulator or the design of the simulation. If not anticipated, gaps in action fidelity can undermine the psychological fidelity of a simulation

■ *Environmental fidelity* involves the setting in which the simulation takes place. Although highest when simulations are played in situ, adequate levels of environmental fidelity may be established in the laboratory. Data from research demonstrate that learner recall and application of content from simulation is highest when it is taught and rehearsed in contexts similar to real life or the workplace (National Research Council, 2000)

■ *Psychological fidelity*, according to Khan et al. (2011), describes simulation's ability to evoke in participants "suspension of disbelief," their willingness to accept the scenario as "real" and, as a consequence, to faithfully perform across several domains (cognitive, psychomotor, and affective) in the simulated environment just as they would in the actual patient care environment. Psychological fidelity is directly influenced by the characteristics of the individual(s) playing the simulation, including his or her perceptions of the simulation (i.e., participant "buy-in" along with personal and professional attributes) and attention to, and faithful reproduction of, action and environmental fidelities. Along with mechanical (equipment) fidelity, psychological fidelity is a major contributor to the perception fidelity of a scenario

■ *Temporal fidelity* refers to the recreation of events along a realistic timeline, as they would occur during actual patient care. One example of adherence to temporal fidelity is delaying the availability of results of laboratory tests ordered during a simulation as experienced in real-life scenarios. Along with mechanical (equipment) fidelity and psychological fidelity, temporal fidelity is a third major contributor to the perception fidelity of a scenario

As these considerations should make clear, the degree of perception fidelity is not merely a function of the mechanical fidelity of a simulator. The receptivity of the learner to the simulation, the learner's reaction, comprehension, and interpretation of actual and perceived stimuli experienced during a simulation, also heavily influence the level of fidelity of the simulated event. We use this to our advantage when designing simulations. To create in the learner the perception of a "complex" situation does not usually require elaborate case development. One or two well-positioned design elements are usually enough to "dazzle the eye" and "confound the intellect" of the learner. In addition, it is often impossible to maintain high levels of fidelity in all of the areas mentioned above. Temporal fidelity is a prime example. In our program, as in most EM programs, most cases last no longer than approximately 10 to 15 minutes. The true-to-life play of a complex case, which would normally require hours to unfold, is just not possible in this time frame. We acknowledge this and most learners accept it. Effective scenario engineering and maintenance of high levels of psychological, perceptual, and action fidelities can overcome a diminished level of temporal fidelity.

FIDELITY MANAGEMENT AND SCENARIO DEVELOPMENT

Awareness of and attention to fidelity in simulation is known as fidelity management. Although "the subjectiveness of fidelity makes fidelity management complex" (Khan et al., 2011), it is nonetheless required if faculty are to expect meaningful learning to occur as a result. Learning with SBE has been shown to occur best when the situation has high perception fidelity (Issenberg et al., 2005; Motola et al., 2013) and is coupled with immediate feedback. The various evidence-based features of simulations that have been demonstrated to foster a high degree of perception fidelity, and which we are careful to include in the design of our simulation-based instruction, aim to:

- develop authentic cases, including genuine and accurate presentations and depictions of conditions, illnesses, and injuries
- provide realistic patient-specific details (e.g., age, sex, personality, socio-economic status, etc.)
- moulage manikins and standardized actors to realistically assist in condition and injury portrayal
- prepare the environment to conform to reality
- provide authentic consequences to the decisions taken and actions performed (or not)
- create complex situations and circumstances, in keeping with individual session-specific goals and objectives
- embed standardized actors, and use these well-trained, scripted confederates whenever possible (in preference to clinical faculty or department staff members, unless their inclusion is essential to meet case- or session-related goals and objectives); and, perhaps most importantly of all
- to establish a "fiction contract" with EM residents, other health professions learners, standardized confederate actors, and all others involved in the portrayal of the simulated patient encounter, to maintain psychological fidelity as if within the actual environment

STRATEGIES FOR ADULT LEARNERS

Overall considerations in designing SBE adhere to the basic educational strategies previously outlined with respect to deliberate practice: (1) to promote experiential learning, described by Kolb (1984) and Kolb and Kolb (2005), as a preferred instructional strategy for adult learners (e.g., active experimentation, reflection on concrete experience, observation, and abstract conceptualization) and (2) to treat mistakes and errors during simulations as mysteries or "puzzles" that need to be solved. Risks of reprimand, of "failing the case," or of consequences resulting from high-stakes assessment do not exist in SBE. Although simulation does have a role in high-stakes, summative assessment, and we do use it for these purposes, we employ SBE strictly for formative assessment. When we perform high-stakes assessments using simulation, the activity ceases to be SBE.

TABLE 6.3 Characteristics of Adult Learners

Are internally motivated and self-directed; need to be involved in the planning and evaluation of their instruction
Like to be respected; possess a deep psychological need to be perceived by others as being self-directed
Bring life experiences and knowledge to learning experiences; experiences (including mistakes) provide a rich basis for learning; experiences provide a framework upon which to anchor new concepts and skills; experiences define who the learners are
Are goal-oriented; need to understand why it is important to learn something; want to apply tomorrow what has been learned today
Learn best when topics are relevant (e.g., of immediate value) or directly related to their jobs or personal lives; educational interests reflect vocational concerns; motivation for learning is increasingly the product of the need to develop knowledge/skills required for performance of evolving societal roles (e.g., medical student training to become a physician)
Are practical; tend to have a problem-centered orientation, not a content-centered orientation, to learning
Have pre-established learning styles; very strong resistance to change

Adapted from Knowles (1973, 1980).

We also try to design our simulation-based experiences to appeal to the unique characteristics of our learners. Current EM residents are clearly both adult learners and millennials, as described by Knowles (1973, 1984) and Roberts, Newman, and Schwartzstein (2012). The features of adult learners and millennials are described in Tables 6.3 and 6.4, respectively. We embrace several of these traits, and try to leverage them, when designing our simulations. For example, adult learners prefer to learn material that is immediately relevant to their job-related tasks; they "want to apply tomorrow what they have learned today." We focus SBE content, therefore, on "high-yield" material that, generally speaking, is almost always linked to the EM Model, with an emphasis on two specific content types: (1) typical and atypical presentations of high frequency conditions, illnesses, and injuries, with an emphasis on high acuity in complex, atypical circumstances; and (2) typical and atypical presentations of high acuity, life- or limb-threatening conditions, illnesses, and injuries, with an emphasis on low-frequency events. We also know that adult learners prefer to use previously developed frameworks, based on and developed through past experience and knowledge, as foundations upon which to layer new knowledge and experiences. Our SBE scenarios for more advanced EM residents are therefore considerably more complex than those tailored for novice learners, and they build on "illness scripts" already formed and catalogued through simulated and actual clinical experience. Cases vary in range of difficulty, and we craft them to portray the continuum of variation that residents may expect to encounter in the actual patient care environment.

Regarding millennial learners, we know that they prefer educational experiences with a problem-centered approach that promotes critical thinking and incorporates synthesis, application, analysis, reasoning, interpretation, and

TABLE 6.4 Characteristics of Millennial Learners

Racially and ethnically diverse; more likely to have experienced racial segregation in previous educational settings/neighborhoods; ambitious; confident; wealthier
Need guidance and focus in their learning (especially when using the internet to search for evidence-based information); require faculty to help them prioritize and identify context for their learning; "pressured" and perhaps overwhelmed by the volume, magnitude, power, and accessibility of information available through technology (e.g., Internet, smart phones)
Will likely use current eLearning technologies to study both independently or collaboratively
Value and expect aesthetically appealing, entertaining, and engaging educational presentations/experiences; prefer to apply knowledge through problems that require critical thinking; prefer a problem-centered approach to learning (in contrast to a "content-centered" approach) that incorporates synthesis, application, analysis, reasoning, interpretation, and other more complex thinking and processing
Are curious and motivated to learn, but may demonstrate "more modern" approaches of exploration or forms of creative thinking; require faculty, at times, to focus on the outcomes of educational experiences, and not processes used to obtain the outcomes
Often more comfortable working and collaborating in groups; are team oriented
Demonstrate less patience with delays; expect resources and support to be available "on-demand," asynchronously, and during "off-hours;" demonstrate a sense of being "special," "sheltered," and "self-confident"
Expect transparency from faculty (clearly defined goals and objectives, useful and meaningful feedback); expect learning to occur in an environment that is fair, impartial, unbiased, and reasonable (no "midstream" rule changes)

Adapted from Roberts et al. (2012).

other types of complex information processing, especially within teams and involving collaboration (Roberts et al., 2012). We therefore structure SBE to match experiences for our EM residents in the actual environment. Just as they rarely provide patient care alone in real life, residents participate in simulations in interprofessional teams, and mixed levels of learners are placed together with nurses and, when possible, with practitioners of other disciplines. Senior residents are given the opportunity to practice attending-level skills; junior residents are allowed more advanced privileges, responsibilities, and significantly greater autonomy than is usually possible in the actual environment. Case management requires collaboration and cooperation. As described earlier, the cases used for these high-fidelity, high-technology simulations are structured to focus on critical thinking, teamwork, situational awareness, and medical decision making in complex situations with layered challenges. The range of difficulty of the cases we select, and the clinical variation we attempt to capture, are rather high in order to meet the expectations of our adult millennial learners.

The final feature of our simulation program, which we view as essential for success, is its integration within the overall EMRP curriculum. SBE is most successful and provides the greatest benefit when it forms part of a larger, overarching curriculum in which simulation is an educational strategy designated to deliver select components and meet specific goals and objectives (Khan et al., 2011; Motola et al., 2013). A number of program-related, institutional, and health system-specific factors influence SBE integration. As the majority of simulation-based experiences for the NS-LIJ EMRP involve high-fidelity, high-technology simulation at PSI, we focus our description below on that portion of the curriculum; but we should note that significant SBE experiences occur as sessions embedded within the didactic conference, including those at the BioSkills Center, and others occur asynchronously, such as in-situ multidisciplinary interprofessional trauma simulations.

SCENARIO DESIGN

EMRP simulation experiences at PSI are 3-hour, small-group afternoon sessions that take place after 5 hours of ACGME-mandated didactic conferences; up to six residents are assigned to participate in the weekly sessions. Each group is assigned to participate in a minimum of two, and a maximum of three, high-fidelity simulations, depending on the complexity of cases to be played. Each hour usually consists of at least one simulation that lasts, on average, 10 minutes and a debriefing that may take at least 40 minutes. During each simulation, a team of at least two but no more than three members cares for the patient. If the group for the week has more than three members, it is divided into two smaller subgroups, each with at least two members. When there are two teams, we use one of two formats. In one format, identical cases play out in consecutive 10-minute intervals for each team (with teams blinded to each other's performance), followed by an immediate combined debriefing. The other format involves two cases with initially identical stems but terminally divergent etiologies; each team plays one case and watches the other. We describe this second model as "compare and contrast," and use it specifically to allow learners to experience twice as much content, to learn vicariously (watching and being in association with others, as described by Lave & Wegner, 1991), as well as through active participation (consistent with Kolb, 1984; Kolb & Kolb, 2005), and to debrief conditions within one domain that appear similar but require distinctively different management. Regardless of the model, EMRP simulation experiences are planned, organized educational events that fulfill a curricular purpose; they are expected and scheduled events, not random, "add-on" supplemental sessions; they are fully integrated into the curriculum.

As an embedded andragogy within our curriculum, we align our program directly with the content covered in the weekly didactic educational sessions. The weekly program is divided into 18 separate modules, each lasting 1 calendar month. All content derives from the EM Model (described previously), which consists of the same number of separate listings of conditions and disease. Within each domain, we choose only the portions specifically requiring SBE as the basis for simulation. We believe this maintains an appropriate level of integration between the overall didactic curriculum and simulation-specific content; to indiscriminately apply simulation as an educational strategy for all components within each domain when other methods are equally effective would be a misallocation of resources. We believe every educational strategy has its appropriate application (even lecture-based instruction); we aim to use each one judiciously.

To summarize, we incorporate the following design elements when structuring our SBE experiences:

- immediate feedback (case play-specific as provided by the simulator, and debriefing-specific as provided by the faculty moderating the simulation)
- high-perception fidelity (acknowledging the interplay between all forms of fidelity that contribute to overall perception fidelity)
- integration with the overarching EMRP curriculum

We usually prepare simulation sessions so that one team of residents manages one patient per scenario. We design the scenarios to follow one of two models: a linear pathway with minimal variation along which the progression of events is sequential, or a branching pathway in which the progression of events may be sequential but accommodates individual team-specific variability. Linear scenarios are useful for assessment of performance concerning conditions for which we expect a minimum level of competency. Branching scenarios allow us to follow more closely the diagnostic and therapeutic paths and to individualize the flow of the case.

PROBLEM IDENTIFICATION AND TARGETED NEEDS ASSESSMENT

When we design simulation cases, we start by thinking about the educational problems we are attempting to solve and how they fit within the overall curriculum. Often these problems revolve around specific gaps (sometimes referred to as "deltas") between ideal and actual performance. We classify these performance gaps using the six domains for clinical medical competence established by the ACGME: patient care, medical knowledge, practice-based learning and improvement, interpersonal and communication skills, professionalism, and systems-based practice. We attempt to identify all the domain-specific deficiencies that we believe constitute etiologies for performance gaps before proceeding to session design and case development, because they directly inform and influence our goals, objectives, and educational strategies. Deficiencies in medical knowledge or technical skill proficiency, common sources for performance gaps seen among EM residents, often require completely different approaches and debriefing styles; these must be considered during the planning stage.

Simulation has been used to help narrow performance gaps in all six ACGME performance domains, including those considered by many to be the most difficult to improve: professionalism and interpersonal and communication skills. These are often the easiest to identify, and medical educators are likely most comfortable with designing education focused on correcting and improving knowledge and performance in these areas. We consciously try, however, to consider all other domains of performance where improvement may be needed, such as nontechnical skills and professional characteristics. "Medical education has traditionally favored mastery of factual knowledge over experiential learning, though there is a notable shift toward a more balanced approach that recognizes both as providing important and complementary cognitive resources." (Cooke, Irby, and O'Brien, 2010, p. 46). Such a shift in perspective recognizes that medical knowledge is "distributed throughout the clinical environment," creating a framework for safety and quality improvement.

GOALS AND OBJECTIVES

In designing simulations, medical educators face important questions concerning choice of content and evaluation of accordance with its goals and objectives. How do we identify important content to be covered over the course of a 3-hour session? And how do we confirm that residents are learning the content we claim to expose them to? These are important questions to answer, as "simulation in the absence of a well thought-out scenario with defined educational goals and objectives is rarely as effective as a well-planned, well-executed event" (Issenberg et al., 2005). Once these are established and agreed upon, and we are sure they align with the EM Model (curricular integration), we can then begin to formulate the scenario; this is sometimes referred to as scenario engineering (Khan et al., 2011).

We start with a base scenario that includes several essential elements that form the foundation of the case, including the patient's diagnosis or diagnoses and the etiology of those conditions, illnesses, or injuries. We briefly describe the patient's physical appearance, initial vital signs, and presenting complaint(s); the relevant history and background story (context) and onset of symptoms; findings on physical examination; and other relevant features such as the patient's socioeconomic status, personality, beliefs, attitudes, language, mental status, and so on. Around these foundations we develop the specific materials to establish the patient's identity, including visual stimuli (electrocardiographs, radiographs), documents (medical records), moulage (bruises, wounds, scars), and props (glasses, wigs, clothes). In addition, we incorporate "case modifiers"—that is, specific design elements not necessary or germane to the case, which we superimpose to enhance fidelity and complexity. These modifications, which we use for more-advanced learners, include language barriers, sensory impairments, and physical or mental impediments (e.g., aphasia). We may also include contextual nuances (such as domestic violence or latent safety threats) or specific settings (e.g., a community-based emergency department setting vs. a tertiary, academic unit).

When we modify a case to incorporate technical skills, we often change the design to form a hybrid in which simulations combine two or more modalities within a single session. The combinations we use most often in our program are high-fidelity simulation using a computer-enhanced manikin simulator and a partial task trainer or a standardized confederate actor.

One special set of case modifiers that we always include in our session design and scenario engineering consists of five basic, evidence-based patient safety-centric behaviors, included by agreement with the PSI: handwashing, self/team identification, patient identification (using two separate identifiers), donning/doffing of personal protective equipment (where appropriate), and using effective team-based/patient-centered communication techniques (e.g., closed-loop communication). These five behaviors form and support a basic "hidden curriculum" in patient safety that is also laid upon the base scenario and superimposed case modifiers.

The selection of the base scenario and various case modifiers depends upon the goals and objectives for the session and the case; they must be strategically aligned, together with the safety-related behaviors, to support the curriculum. Once faculty are comfortable that all elements are in place, the case is written. We use a modified case template incorporating others previously described by McLaughlin et al. (2008), Alinier (2010), and others (Association of American Medical Colleges, 2009; Seropian, Brown, Gavilanes, & Driggers, 2004). This framework is consistent with the generally accepted methods of instructional design and includes the scenario title, target audience, goals and objectives (including case-specific "critical actions"), case narrative (including chief complaints, history of present illness, past history, medications, allergies, social and family histories, and advance directives), physical examination, scenario-specific instructor notes (including case play, branching or linear flow diagrams, critical action checklists and other evaluation forms/rubrics), stimuli, design notes (case premieres, authorship), reflections (we refer to them as deltas) derived from pilot testing and actual implementation, and, finally, references providing the evidence basis. To this scenario template we attach a session lesson plan, complete with faculty and student guides that corresponds to the scenarios within the session.

At times, the curriculum places unique demands upon the SBE experience. Curricular goals and objectives, for example, might require that EM residents demonstrate the ability to contemporaneously manage several patients at once. In such cases we incorporate novel session design and scenario engineering (e.g., "Sim ED," Nemes et al., 2013) to create a simulation strategy to meet these unique demands.

SUMMARY

Simulation plays an expanding and ever more integral role in the education and assessment of today's EM residents. For adult millennial medical learners, SBE appears more effective than other strategies for imparting to residents the knowledge, attitudes, and requisite skills for safe patient care and multidisciplinary, interprofessional collaborative practice; it also responds to the mandate of external stakeholders for more robust learner assessments. As the evolution of our program indicates, the future holds promise for greater complexity, fidelity, and sophistication in instructional design.

NOTE

1. Laerdal Medical Corporation, Wappingers Falls, New York. The purchase was funded in part by a grant obtained by Joseph LaMantia and Michael Cassara through the Geriatrics for Specialists Initiative, co-sponsored by the American Geriatrics Society and John A. Hartford Foundation.

REFERENCES

Accreditation Council for Graduate Medical Education & the American Board of Medical Specialties. (2000). *Toolbox of assessment methods: A product of the Joint Initiative ACGME Outcome Project* (1.1 ed., pp. 13–14). http://www.dconnect.acgme.org/outcome/assess/toolbox.asp

Aggarwal, R., Grantcharov, T., & Darzi, A. (2007). Framework for systematic training and assessment of technical skills. *Journal of the American College of Surgeons, 204*(4), 697–705. doi:10.1016/j.jamcollsurg.2007.01.016

Alinier, G. (2010). Developing high-fidelity health care simulation scenarios: A guide for educators and professionals. *Simulation & Gaming, 42*(1), 9–26. doi:10.1177/1046878109355683

American Board of Emergency Medicine. (2013). *History of the American Board of Emergency Medicine.* Retrieved from https://www.abem.org/public/general-information/history

American College of Emergency Physicians. (2008). *Definition of emergency medicine.* Retrieved from http://www.acep.org/content.aspx?id=29164

Association of American Medical Colleges. (2009). *Human patient simulation template.* Retrieved from https://www.mededportal.org/download/191144/data/human_patient_simulation_case_template.pdf

Cantrell, M. A. (2008). The importance of debriefing in clinical simulations. *Clinical Simulation in Nursing, 4*(2), e19–e23. doi:10.1016/j.ecns.2008.06.006

Cooke, M., Irby, D. M., & O'Brien C. (2010). *Educating Physicians: A Call for Reform of Medical School and Residency.* San Francisco: Jossey Bass.

Dreifuerst, K. T. (2009). The essentials of debriefing in simulation learning: A concept analysis. *Nursing Education Perspectives, 30*(2), 109–114.

Ericsson, K. A. (Ed.). (2009). *Development of professional expertise: Toward measurement of expert performance and design of optimal learning environments.* New York, NY: Cambridge University Press.

Fanning, R. M., & Gaba, D. M. (2007). The role of debriefing in simulation-based learning. *Simulation in Healthcare, 2*(2), 115–125.

Issenberg, S. B., McGaghie, W. C., Petrusa, E. R., Lee Gordon, D., & Scalese, R. J. (2005). Features and uses of high-fidelity medical simulations that lead to effective learning: A BEME systematic review. *Medical Teacher, 27*(1), 10–28. doi:10.1080/01421590500046924

Khan, K., Tolhurst-Cleaver, S., White, S., & Simpson, W. (2011). Simulation in healthcare education: Building a simulation programme: A practical guide. In T. Gibbs (Series Ed.), *AMEE guide series 2* (Vol. 50, p. 44). Dundee, UK: Association for Medical Educators in Europe.

Knowles, M. S. (1973). *The adult learner: A neglected species.* Houston, TX: Gulf.

Knowles, M. S. (1980). *The modern practice of adult education: From pedagogy to andragogy (Revised and updated).* New York, NY: The Adult Education.

Knowles, M. (1984). The Adult Learner: A Neglected Species (3rd Ed.). Houston, TX: Gulf Publishing.

Kohn, L. T., Corrigan, J., & Donaldson, M. S. (2000). *To err is human: Building a safer health system.* Washington, DC: National Academy Press.

Kolb, A., & Kolb, D. (2005). Learning styles and learning spaces: Enhancing experiential learning in higher education. *Academy of Management Learning & Education, 4*(2), 193–212.

Kolb, D. (1984). *Experiential learning: Experience as the source of learning and development.* Englewood Cliffs, NJ: Prentice-Hall.

Lake, F., & Hamdorf, J. (2004). Teaching on the run tips 5: Teaching a skill. *Medical Journal of Australia, 181*(6), 327–328.

Lave, J., & Wenger, E. (1991). *Situated learning: Legitimate peripheral participation* (1st ed.). Cambridge, UK: Cambridge University.

McLaughlin, S., Bond, W., Promes, S., & Spillane, L. (2006). The status of human simulation training in emergency medicine residency programs. *Simulation in Healthcare, 1*(Inaugural), 18–21.

McLaughlin, S., Fitch, M. T., Goyal, D. G., Hayden, E., Yang Kauh, C., Laack, T. A., . . . Gordon, J. A. (2008). Simulation in graduate medical education 2008: A review for emergency medicine. *Academic Emergency Medicine, 15*(11), 1117–1129. doi:10.1111/j.1553-2712.2008.00188.x

Motola, I., Devine, L. A., Chung, H. S., Sullivan, J. E., & Issenberg, S. B. (2013). Simulation in healthcare education: A best evidence practical guide. AMEE Guide No. 82. *Medical Teacher, 35*(10), e1511–e1530. doi:10.3109/0142159X.2013.818632

National Research Council. (2000). *How people learn: Brain, mind, experience, and school: Expanded edition.* Washington, DC: The National Academies Press.

Nemes, P. C., Marcus, D., Sandalow, N., Cassara, M., Farina, G., DeVoe, B., . . . Silverman, R. (2013, September 9). *Sim ED – A simulated emergency department (ED) for teaching and assessing resident communication, multitasking and handoff.* Paper presented at the VIIth Mediterranean Emergency Medicine Congress, Marseille, France.

Noeller, T. P., Smith, M. D., Holmes, L., Cappaert, M., Gross, A. J., Cole-Kelly, K., & Rosen, K. R. (2008). A theme-based hybrid simulation model to train and evaluate emergency medicine residents. *Academic Emergency Medicine, 15*(11), 1199–1206. doi:10.1111/j.1553-2712.2008.00183.x

Okuda, Y., Bond, W., Bonfante, G., McLaughlin, S., Spillane, L., Wang, E., . . . Gordon, J. A. (2008). National growth in simulation training within emergency medicine residency programs, 2003–2008. *Academic Emergency Medicine, 15*(11), 1113–1116. doi:10.1111/j.1553-2712.2008.00195.x

Perina, D. G., Brunett C. P., Caro, D. A., Char., D. M., Chisholm, C. D., Counselman, F. L., . . . Ma, O. J. (2012). The 2011 model of the clinical practice of emergency medicine. *Academic Emergency Medicine, 19*(7), e19–e40. doi:10.1111/j.1553-2712.2012.01385.x

Peyton, J. W. R. (1998). The learning cycle. In J. W. R. Peyton (Ed.), *Teaching and learning in medical practice* (pp. 13–19). Rickmansworth, UK: Manticore Europe.

Roberts, D., Newman, L., & Schwartzstein, R. (2012). Twelve tips for facilitating millennials' learning. *Medical Teacher, 34*(4), 274–278. doi:10.3109/0142159X.2011.613498

Seropian, M. A., Brown, K., Gavilanes, J. S., & Driggers, B. (2004). Simulation: Not just a manikin. *Journal of the Nursing Education, 43*(4), 164–169.

Society for Academic Emergency Medicine. (2014). Retrieved from http://beta.saem.org/membership/services/residency-directory

Swing, S. (2002). Assessing the ACGME general competencies: General considerations and assessment methods. *Academic Emergency Medicine, 9*(11), 1278–1288.

Van de Ridder, J. M., Stokking, K. M., McGaghie, W. C., & ten Cate, O. T. (2008). What is feedback in clinical education? *Medical Education, 42*(2), 189–197. doi:10.1111/j.1365-2923.2007.02973.x

Van Heukelom, J. N., Begaz, T., & Treat, R. (2010). Comparison of post-simulation debriefing versus in-simulation debriefing in medical simulation. *Simulation in Healthcare, 5*(2), 91–97. doi:10.1097/SIH.0b013e3181be0d17

Wang, E., Quinones, J., Fitch, M., Dooley-Hash, S., Griswold-Theodorson, S., Medzon, R., . . . Clay, L. (2008). Developing technical expertise in emergency medicine—the role of simulation in procedural skill acquisition. *Academic Emergency Medicine, 15*(11), 1046–1057. doi: 10.1111/j.1553-2712.2008.00218.x

Three: Pediatric and Perinatal Interprofessional Teams

Leah Kaufman
Adiel Fleisher
M. Isabel Friedman
Robert L. Kerner Jr.

7: Essential Maneuvers: Simulation as Part of a Long-Term Comprehensive Perinatal Safety Initiative

A comprehensive program to improve patient safety in a regional perinatal center that delivers more than 5,000 infants annually employed simulation as an integral component of enhanced teamwork and communication with a view to reducing adverse outcomes and avoiding interventions that risk unnecessary complications. In addition to high-fidelity simulation, the ongoing program has developed realistic scenarios and uses standardized patients to help caregivers practice and improve disclosure of adverse events in ways that meet the needs of patients, their families, and caregivers themselves.

In the perinatal setting, simulation can play multiple roles to help achieve the high degree of safety we require. Obstetrics is a specialty in which a great many situations rely on special maneuvers that are complex and difficult, if not impossible, to teach in a classroom. Many of the unpredictable complications of childbirth, such as shoulder dystocia and placental abruption, must be treated as emergencies and carry the risk of lifelong disability and even death. In addition, procedures in the perinatal setting demand a true team effort that cannot be developed by individuals learning in silos; simulation provides the opportunity for interprofessional, experiential learning. For patients, emotions and expectations run extremely high and disappointment with anything less than perfection can provoke corresponding dissatisfaction and reproach, with both psychological and potentially legal consequences for caregivers. For all these reasons, to put it succinctly, "Obstetrics is the ideal field in which to apply simulation training" (Deering, 2008).

As a regional perinatal center that delivers more than 5,000 infants each year, we are a tertiary facility with an estimated 20% to 30% of our obstetrics patients at elevated or high risk for complications. In late 2005 we began to develop a simulation program in collaboration with the newly opened Patient Safety Institute (PSI) at North Shore-LIJ (NS-LIJ). Soon thereafter, we designed and subsequently reported on a comprehensive perinatal safety initiative that we implemented stepwise over the course of 2 years, beginning in 2007 (Wagner et al., 2012). Simulation formed one central feature of this initiative, which we used in multiple ways to address adverse outcomes, improve teamwork, and teach communications skills.

STIMULUS FROM WITHIN AND WITHOUT

Both growing attention to patient safety in obstetrics and internal events at our hospital disposed us to action. As was the case with similar efforts elsewhere (Pratt et al., 2007), sentinel events and near misses prompted us to undertake a root cause analysis—that is, a case-based review of system failures (Grunebaum, 2007; Mann & Pratt, 2008). Broader impetus, we should add, arose from growing concern about safety in the obstetrics community. The 1999 watershed Institute of Medicine report and subsequent publications raised awareness throughout the health care community (Institute of Medicine Committee on Quality of Health Care in America, 2001; Kohn, Corrigan, & Donaldson, 2000); there were also recommendations in 2003 from the American College of Obstetricians and Gynecologists (ACOG) and discussions of "another national malpractice crisis in obstetrics" (American College of Obstetricians and Gynecologists [ACOG], 2003; Kohn et al., 2000). Although progress in most specialties turned out to be slow, as Leape and Berwick emphasized in an overview 5 years after publication of *To Err Is Human*, the problem of patient safety was beginning to engage perinatal medicine, just as in the previous decade it had brought about significant and quantifiable changes in anesthesiology (Leape & Berwick, 2005). We became one of many perinatal health centers in the United States to raise safety awareness in the first decade of the 21st century, and one of several to quantify improvement with a comprehensive safety initiative (DuPree, O'Neill, & Anderson, 2009).

Results of our internal and external audit, in retrospect, not surprisingly aligned with a widely disseminated 2004 report from The Joint Commission that pointed to failures in communication as the underlying cause of up to 80% of adverse and near-harm events (Scalise, 2006). A single assessor, after performing monthly evaluations of all obstetrical hemorrhage charts and 10 charts with abnormal fetal heart rate (FHR) tracings, identified four causes of adverse events: poor communication among providers, inadequate escalation policies, insufficient protocols, and lack of standards for interpreting FHR tracings. It was in light of these findings that we established an interdisciplinary perinatal safety committee whose members included physicians, nurses, educators, and administrators. It was charged with developing and implementing the various components of the initiative, including several measures for assessment of outcomes over time.

Inauguration of daily working rounds each morning constituted our first step in what we envisaged from the start as a broader initiative. These rounds were interdisciplinary and included, at a minimum, the attending physician (as team leader), a subspecialist in neonatal medicine, the unit resident, a physician assistant, the nursing staff (including the supervisor for labor and delivery), and the anesthesiologist. The team attended to every patient, reviewing and discussing any and all relevant issues concerning assessment, management, and plans of action, including any special issues or risk factors that might call for escalation; and we sought to enhance awareness of potential "hot" situations that could require additional personnel or resources.

We also instituted several educational components. Our adoption of the Team Strategies and Tools to Enhance Performance and Patient Safety (Team-STEPPS®) targeted both training methods and daily procedures on the floor of the perinatal unit (King et al., 2008). Equally helpful was a comprehensive course on interpretation and management of FHR patterns that covered the definitions, pathophysiology, clinical relevance of changes, and significance with respect to fetal oxygenation, fetal acid base values, and management scenarios. A chief goal here, as elsewhere, was to improve communication by eliminating discrepancies in terminology and procedures. Every member of the team—including nurses, residents, and attending physicians—had to complete the same course and take the same exam. We achieved full compliance.

In addition, we inaugurated no fewer than seven new or revised evidence-based protocols. They included use of Pitocin (oxytocin) to induce labor, and we empowered any team member to cite this protocol and act on it when presented with an abnormal FHR tracing. We introduced rules governing induction of labor, management of FHR abnormalities, the assembly and behavior of a rapid response team, use of antibiotics, thromboembolic prophylaxis for cesarean births, and administration of magnesium to prevent seizures.

High-Fidelity Simulation for the Acute Emergency

Our work with simulation predated the safety initiative, evolved in conjunction with it, and continues today as part of a long-term effort to address specific high-risk albeit low-frequency emergencies and, more broadly but no less significantly, to improve team communication and quality of care. Among the various options, we had recourse to the Center for Learning and Innovation (CLI), our corporate university, and its Patient Safety Institute (PSI), an external simulation facility around which we could organize curricula; we made use of the flexibility these resources provided to shape specific scenarios and tasks both for teams and individual learners, with a view to improving overall performance and the treatment of specific low-frequency emergencies.

We developed our first simulation scenarios in 2006, focusing on some of the sentinel events in our hospital; similar events were at the same time also manifest and much-discussed concerns of the obstetrics community nationwide (Mann & Pratt, 2008). Catastrophic hemorrhage, seizure, hypertensive emergency, and shoulder dystocia were early and durable examples. For each, we developed a set of presimulation materials and conducted brief didactics that included basic information, distribution of canonical articles, and a pretest. All teams were multidisciplinary, including nursing staff and residents or physician assistants, with the attending physician observing from the control room and monitoring simulation sessions. As it developed over time, PSI (which also enlarged and enhanced its services) provided dedicated nursing personnel to orient participants, including a clinical specialist to act as an adjunct facilitator in the debriefing sessions. Our videotaped simulations in these contexts used the full-size birthing manikin NOELLE®,[1] and we started to typically run several six-member teams during a single simulation.

Shoulder dystocia, the unpredictable emergency during childbirth that requires rapid recognition and specific maneuvers to complete delivery, represents a good example of a sentinel event for high-fidelity simulation (Crofts et al., 2008). Estimates of its frequency vary, as reported in the literature, from 0.2% to 3% of vaginal deliveries (Grobman, 2013); several risk factors (previous shoulder dystocia, maternal diabetes, prolonged second stage of labor, birth weight, and others) can be identified but none are usefully predictive. If not properly and promptly addressed, shoulder dystocia can result in brachial plexus injuries or fetal hypoxic injury; there is the risk of lifelong disability and even death. For these reasons, shoulder dystocia is characterized as an obstetrical nightmare and "[f]ew obstetric emergencies cause as much anxiety" (Fahey & Mighty, 2008, p. 121). In line with recommendations of The Joint Commission and the gathering consensus around safety concerns in the obstetrical community, we developed a simulation curriculum for this uncommon but not rare emergency ("Sentinel event alert issue 30–July 21, 2004. Preventing infant death and injury during delivery," 2004).

For this high-fidelity simulation, we ordinarily begin sessions with the nurse, who discovers the patient—the full-size manikin—in pain and ready to push. In addition to remotely manipulating vital signs, including contraction pattern and FHR, we provide the voice of the patient from the control booth. Based on her communication with the patient, the nurse is expected to call for a resident (or advanced practice provider). We observe their history taking and their assessment of the patient's risk factors as well as team communication.

When the delivery begins, the infant's head emerges but the shoulder remains lodged despite gentle downward traction. We expect the resident to call for help, announce the diagnosis of shoulder dystocia to the team, and begin to perform the maneuvers to dislodge the baby and complete the delivery. Most deliveries succeed after several attempts. As we observe and, acting as the voice of the patient, continuously communicate with the team, we have the ability to respond to the teamwork dynamic, to change the scenario and make the delivery more challenging. A variety of factors influence our decision as to when to conclude the scenario, which might include a post-delivery conversation to explain the birth complication in nontechnical terms to the mother.

Debriefings for shoulder dystocia normally last much longer than the simulations themselves. They richly engage learners on several distinct levels. Due to the fact that we do not interfere with the simulation while it is in progress, the debrief represents the key stage of learning and assimilation. Participants are encouraged to provide an orderly account of the case and evaluate their own actions while the facilitator—an attending physician and a debriefing expert—ensure that the learning objectives are met. Importantly, caregivers' knowledge of the medicine and underlying science should align with their cognitive understanding of the situation and with the actions they took. This is the place to address gaps in knowledge, skills, and attitude. As a complication of pregnancy that interrupts normal progress to delivery and suddenly transforms it into an acute emergency, shoulder dystocia provokes anxiety and powerfully challenges team communication. Debriefs allow team members to decompress, engage in self-discovery and reflection, express how they were feeling, examine their interactions with one another and with the patient, and effectively practice for the future.

Participants complete the shoulder dystocia simulation with a posttest and they also develop record-keeping notes that chronicle and document details of the delivery.

Disclosure of Adverse Events With Standardized Patients

For shoulder dystocia and other delivery room emergencies, we also developed simulation activities that aim to help clinicians and teams learn how to deliver "bad news" to parents and family members. While adverse outcomes are uncommon in the perinatal setting, they are inevitable. Mother and family deserve a sensitive response, and explanations of clinical decisions, including the science that underlies and supports them, in ordinary language. Caregivers should offer genuine expressions of empathy and counseling with attention to providing explanation and not attributing blame to individuals.

In medicine, only in recent years has significant attention been paid to issues around disclosure of bad news—indeed, owing in part to the developing patient safety movement with its emphasis on the patient's autonomy and need to know (Conway, 2011). Whether an adverse outcome is unpreventable, unforeseen, or due to iatrogenic error, caregivers must be able to cope with a range of emotional reactions from patients and family members. Lack of interpersonal skills and clumsiness in providing explanations in language that patients can understand readily provoke anger and resentment (Fallowfield & Jenkins, 2004).

As an example of one of many scenarios using standardized patients for disclosure of adverse events, we can continue with shoulder dystocia. The challenge for the caregiver is to explain both the event itself and the adverse outcome clearly, empathically, and without medical jargon. In advance of the session we provide several articles, including ACOG's Committee Opinion on "Disclosure and Discussion of Adverse Events" (Committee on Patient Safety and Quality Improvement, & Committee on Professional Liability, 2012; Cushing & Jones, 1995; Grobman, 2013). Also, we adapted the protocol known as SPIKES (see Chapter 9), a widely used six-step strategy originally designed for oncology that details how to carefully approach and sensitively attend to the patient's perceptions, to provide good information according to his or her needs, and offer a strategy for moving forward (Baile et al., 2000). Risks to caregivers themselves represent another important aspect of disclosure, so for simulation participants we also screen the brief video "Healing Our Own: Adverse Events in Obstetrics and Gynecology" (American College of Obstetricians and Gynecologists, 2012).

Scenario for Disclosure Our scenarios for these counseling simulations aim to rapidly set up recognizable situations. Into each case we build dramatic features with learning objectives. Prior to the session the major facts and details of the case are read aloud to our multidisciplinary team participants. In one, for example, the patient was a 43-year-old woman who presented at labor with spontaneous rupture of membranes and said she felt she would need to push. Her current pregnancy had been uncomplicated and she had previously delivered three full-term infants and had one terminated pregnancy. Infant birth weight was estimated to be 9 pounds, her blood pressure was normal, and she did not suffer from diabetes.

But, we continue to explain to the team, this apparently straightforward delivery did not progress as expected. The patient was initially dilated at 5 to 6 cm and the delivery over the course of an hour progressed to the anterior tip, making an epidural impossible. For 20 minutes she pushed and the baby's head descended to the +3 station; it could be seen without retracting the labia. At that point she said she could push no longer and requested a caesarian: "Just give me a section."

The team replied by encouraging her: "You've delivered a larger baby in the past and you can do it this time, too." She made three further attempts to push and delivered the vertex. But now a shoulder dystocia was noted. The resident called for help and the patient was placed in the McRobert's position. The nurse performed suprapubic pressure. Finally, the anterior right shoulder was dislodged with the help of an episiotomy and the Woods maneuver.

The delivery concluded with an adverse outcome. The infant girl (7.9 Apgar, 10 lbs) had an absent Moro response on the left. Two days after delivery she could not move her left arm and manifested weakness in her left hand. The diagnosis was a left clavicular fracture.

Simulation The team's tasks are several: to answer all questions and to explain to the mother and other family members the circumstances of the delivery, the adverse outcome, and the prognosis.

Either the resident or nurse may enter the room first to find the mother in bed and in the company of a family member. Intentionally, the physical layout of the multi-bed hospital room creates issues that need to be addressed: a second patient is present, necessitating a curtain to be drawn for privacy before discussing the adverse event during delivery. In addition, a chair is placed in a corner of the room so that the resident needs to purposefully move it close to the patient to facilitate eye contact and conversation.

The mother displays distress:

"We just need answers. We don't understand. Everything was okay with my baby. I didn't have any problems. This wasn't supposed to happen. I just want answers."

"I had three babies before this. None of them gave me trouble like this one. Why did this happen? I just want to know."

"Another thing I don't understand. Why was the baby's weight so off? You estimated one thing but that baby came out at 10 pounds. It just seems to me you could know better."

"How did this happen? I felt it was traumatic, if you ask me. Things were chaotic. It seemed like everybody was running around and nobody knew what to do next. That never happened to me before. I had three babies before this and it never happened."

"Can you just tell me how often this happens? I don't get why you just kept pulling on the baby's head. Then you had to cut it out. Why did you just keep pulling?"

The resident or nurse is expected to engage the patient and her family and at some point request help from the team. Body language will be important and the resident or nurse needs to bring a chair closer to the bedside in order not to stand above the patient but, rather, to create a comfortable interpersonal space. Responding to the patient's questions will involve addressing and not evading them, explaining the sequence of events and decisions taken, as well as avoiding jargon while keeping a focus on the underlying science and clinical best practice. Gestures, intonation, and choice of words all convey information that can impact the patient and provide material for discussion in the subsequent debrief. Distinguishing an inadequate explanation from a usefully informative and empathic one, especially with the help of video recordings, does not generally prove difficult:

Inadequate: "To answer your question, you didn't need a C-section. We performed what's known as a McRobert's maneuver and then followed that with suprapubic pressure. But not even that was enough. In the end, we had to perform a minor procedure so you could deliver the baby properly."

Better: "You did fine. Sometimes—not often, but it's not rare, either—the shoulder gets stuck and we have to try some maneuvers. One of them is cutting an episiotomy to dislodge that shoulder and deliver your baby safely. That's what happened."

Debrief The standardized patients who participated in the simulation also attend the debriefing sessions, to help provide feedback by offering their own subjective feelings and reactions to specific caregiver remarks and behavior.

"When you said I didn't need a C-section, I felt like you were insinuating it was my fault."
"Suprapubic pressure? What does that mean?"
"When you said, 'Thank you for your help,' it felt condescending."

Including the standardized patients in the debrief has a further benefit in that team members can immediately practice improved communication. The patient:

"You know, I asked for a C-section. Why didn't you just give me a C-section?"

Instead of the defensive response, "You didn't need a C-section so we couldn't do that," the learner can try out the advocacy/inquisitive model (Rudolph, Simon, Dufresne, & Raemer, 2006):

"I'm curious. Why did you think you needed a C-section?"

Assuming the patient replies along the lines of: "I'd pushed and pushed":

"Sure. I can understand. It seemed like a long time and you were in pain. But at that moment, your delivery was too far along for us to safely give you a C-section."

As in high-fidelity contexts, we have learned to calibrate the challenge in simulations with standardized patients, depending on the perceived skill and experience of individual caregivers. Rather than use a manikin in the room's second bed, we may employ a standardized patient in the role of an intrusive outsider so that confidentiality and diplomacy become issues. Ordinarily, standardized patients are instructed to respond in kind to the caregivers, reflecting empathy or aggression, for example. With experienced caregivers who are well-prepared in disclosing adverse events, we may ask the standardized patient or family member to be accusatory or aggressive under all circumstances.

Outcomes and Aspects of a Safety Culture

Simulation formed a core aspect of the methodology in our patient safety initiative and we did not attempt to separately measure its contribution. Studies have demonstrated the value of high-fidelity simulation for the treatment of shoulder dystocia (Crofts, Winter, & Sowter, 2011), and research also supports the use of standardized patients for this and several other obstetric emergencies (Crofts, Bartlett, et al., 2008). We can, in addition, speak to the question of outcomes more broadly with respect to our perinatal safety initiative, several of its individual components, and perceived measures of improvement in performance and patient satisfaction.

Our primary goal was to improve the quality of care in a large regional perinatal center and to create a culture of patient safety. Research efforts in obstetrics are often constrained by ethical and practical difficulties that make it unfeasible to assign teams to follow different protocols over time; the comparative rarity of adverse outcomes also makes development of validated measures problematic. To that end we adapted the Adverse Outcome Index (AOI), introduced in 2006 by Pratt and colleagues as a set of 13 quality indicators (Mann et al., 2006). We excluded two problematic outcomes (admissions to the neurological intensive care unit and third/fourth degree lacerations), which left 11 measures that we described as the Modified AOI. Cases were logged prospectively after the introduction of the initiative, with the Modified AOI calculated by dividing the number of pregnancies with complications by the total number of deliveries over time. Logistic regression showed that the Modified AOI index rate decreased from 1.95% to 0.89% across calendar year quarters relative to 2007, when the initiative was implemented, before leveling off in 2009. The result was significant ($p < .0004$) and by 2009 represented a 54% decrease in adverse outcomes as measured by the Modified AOI.

We compared our outcomes to other published data, and we also reviewed management and documentation of two high-risk situations: obstetrical hemorrhage and FHR abnormalities. In the absence of a comparative cohort, the contribution of individual components of the perinatal safety initiative could not be easily measured. However, we also evaluated staff perceptions of safety, which showed a positive increase from 2007 to 2009 ($p < .001$) and found nonsignificant improvement in patient perceptions. Our rate of caesarian deliveries did not significantly change, but with respect to FHR abnormalities, the percentage of cases that were appropriately managed increased ($p < .0002$), as did adequate documentation ($p < .0001$).

Iatrogenic Prematurity and a Culture of Patient Safety Although we could not distill the contribution that simulation made to improved outcomes as measured by the Modified AOI, one measure we quantified seems especially worth noting. We virtually eliminated iatrogenic prematurity, with an incidence of 0.2%, far below the target rate of 5% set by The Joint Commission (2013). Although that result could be a statistical outlier, or due to some specific set of protocols, it is also possible that it represents the combined influence and synergistic outcome of algorithms to reduce unnecessary preterm births, to team training, and to simulation. In general, the rate of iatrogenic prematurity at any institution owes to various complications and to demographic and other variables. Positive improvements that affect both team communication and the ability of team members to interact with patients and their families might substantially help reduce it. If validated, such a measure could serve as an indication of the development of a mature safety culture in the perinatal setting.

NOTE

1. Gaumard Scientific. We have since begun to use SimMom® (Laerdal Medical).

REFERENCES

American College of Obstetricians and Gynecologists. (2003). ACOG committee opinion number 286, October 2003: Patient safety in obstetrics and gynecology. *Obstetricians and Gynecologists, 102*(4), 883–885.

American College of Obstetricians and Gynecologists. (2012). *Healing our own: Adverse events in obstetrics and gynecology*. Washington, DC: Author.

Baile, W. F., Buckman, R., Lenzi, R., Glober, G., Beale, E. A., & Kudelka, A. P. (2000). SPIKES—A six-step protocol for delivering bad news: Application to the patient with cancer. *The oncologist, 5*(4), 302–311.

Commission, J. (2013). *Specifications manual for Joint Commission National Quality Measures* (v2013A1). Retrieved from https://manual.jointcommission.org/releases/TJC2013A/MIF0166.html

Committee on Patient Safety and Quality Improvement, & Committee on Professional Liability. (2012). ACOG Committee Opinion No. 520: Disclosure and discussion of adverse events. *Obstetricians and Gynecologists, 119*(3), 686–689. doi:10.1097/AOG.0b013e31824e12f9

Conway, J. F. F., Stewart, K., & Campbell, M. (2011). Respectful management of serious clinical adverse events. In *IHI Innovation Series white paper* (2nd ed.). Cambridge, MA: Institute for Healthcare Improvement.

Crofts, J. F., Bartlett, C., Ellis, D., Winter, C., Donald, F., Hunt, L. P., & Draycott, T. J. (2008). Patient-actor perception of care: A comparison of obstetric emergency training using manikins and patient-actors. *Quality and Safety in Health Care, 17*(1), 20–24. doi:10.1136/qshc.2006.021873

Crofts, J. F., Fox, R., Ellis, D., Winter, C., Hinshaw, K., & Draycott, T. J. (2008). Observations from 450 shoulder dystocia simulations: Lessons for skills training. *Obstetricians and Gynecologists, 112*(4), 906–912. doi:10.1097/AOG.0b013e3181865f55

Crofts, J. F., Winter, C., & Sowter, M. C. (2011). Practical simulation training for maternity care—where we are and where next. *British Journal of Obstetrics and Gynaecology, 118*(Suppl. 3), 11–16. doi:10.1111/j.1471-0528.2011.03175.x

Cushing, A. M., & Jones, A. (1995). Evaluation of a breaking bad news course for medical students. *Medical Education, 29*(6), 430–435.

Deering, S. (2008). Obstetric simulation. In R. H. Riley (Ed.), *Manual of simulation in healthcare* (pp. 351–374). New York, NY: Oxford University Press.

DuPree, E., O'Neill, L., & Anderson, R. M. (2009). Achieving a safety culture in obstetrics. *Mount Sinai Journal of Medicine, 76*(6), 529–538. doi:10.1002/msj.20144

Fahey, J. O., & Mighty, H. E. (2008). Shoulder dystocia: Using simulation to train providers and teams. *The Journal of Perinatal and Neonatal Nursing, 22*(2), 114–122; quiz 123–114. doi:10.1097/01.JPN.0000319097.05415.1d

Fallowfield, L., & Jenkins, V. (2004). Communicating sad, bad, and difficult news in medicine. *Lancet, 363*(9405), 312–319. doi:10.1016/s0140-6736(03)15392-5

Grobman, W. (2013). Shoulder dystocia. *Obstetricians and Gynecologists Clinics of North America, 40*(1), 59–67. doi:10.1016/j.ogc.2012.11.006

Grunebaum, A. (2007). Error reduction and quality assurance in obstetrics. *Clinics in Perinatology, 34*(3), 489–502. doi:10.1016/j.clp.2007.03.017

Institute of Medicine, Committee on Quality of Health Care in America. (2001). *Crossing the quality chasm: A new health system for the 21st century*. Washington, DC: National Academy Press.

King, H. B., Battles, J., Baker, D. P., Alonso, A., Salas, E., Webster, J., . . . Salisbury, M. (2008). *TeamSTEPPS: Team strategies and tools to enhance performance and patient safety*. Rockville, MD: Agency for Healthcare Research and Quality.

Kohn, L. T., Corrigan, J., & Donaldson, M. S. (2000). *To err is human: Building a safer health system*. Washington, DC: National Academy Press.

Leape, L. L., & Berwick, D. M. (2005). Five years after To Err Is Human: What have we learned? *JAMA: The Journal of the American Medical Association, 293*(19), 2384–2390. doi:10.1001/jama.293.19.2384

Mann, S., Pratt, S., Gluck, P., Nielsen, P., Risser, D., Greenberg, P., . . . Sachs, B. (2006). Assessing quality obstetrical care: Development of standardized measures. *Joint Commission Journal on Quality and Patient Safety, 32*(9), 497–505.

Mann, S., & Pratt, S. D. (2008). Team approach to care in labor and delivery. *Clinical Obstetricians and Gynecologists, 51*(4), 666–679. doi:10.1097/GRF.0b013e3181899ac2

Pratt, S. D., Mann, S., Salisbury, M., Greenberg, P., Marcus, R., Stabile, B., . . . Sachs, B. P. (2007). John M. Eisenberg Patient Safety and Quality Awards. Impact of CRM-based training on obstetric outcomes and clinicians' patient safety attitudes. *Joint Commission Journal on Quality and Patient Safety, 33*(12), 720–725.

Rudolph, J. W., Simon, R., Dufresne, R. L., & Raemer, D. B. (2006). There's no such thing as "nonjudgmental" debriefing: A theory and method for debriefing with good judgment. *Simulation in Healthcare, 1*(1), 49–55.

Scalise, D. (2006). Clinical communication and patient safety. *Hospitals and Health Networks, 80*(8), 49–54.

Sentinel event alert issue 30—July 21, 2004. Preventing infant death and injury during delivery. (2004). *Advances in Neonatal Care, 4*(4), 180–181.

Wagner, B., Meirowitz, N., Shah, J., Nanda, D., Reggio, L., Cohen, P., . . . Abrams, K. J. (2012). Comprehensive perinatal safety initiative to reduce adverse obstetric events. *Journal for Healthcare Quality, 34*(1), 6–15. doi:10.1111/j.1945-1474.2011.00134.x

Sandeep Gangadharan
Andrew Rotjan

8: Pediatric Emergencies: Targeted Programs and Crafted Scenarios

The use of simulation in pediatrics to train interprofessional teams constitutes a new paradigm for assessing and managing hospital-based emergencies. Described in this chapter are the ways in which simulation in a tertiary care hospital for children enhances interprofessional education and helps to identify and improve practices, procedures, and policies. Several programs identify and meet specific local needs with a view to discriminate attention to patient safety. These programs are multidisciplinary and provide learners with scenarios that instill all components of efficient response to acute conditions such as severe respiratory failure, sepsis, and change in mental status. Here we describe three of these programs, together with basic concepts underlying scenario construction, using both high-fidelity simulators and standardized patients.

Simulation in pediatrics, as it developed over the past decade, has come to reflect both the specialty's unique challenges and a set of instructive qualities, which may also prove suggestive for wider application in allied and other disciplines. Emphasis on critical care simulation, in particular, owes to the fact that high-risk and low-frequency events, such as airway emergencies and endotracheal intubation, are among the most important contributors to morbidity and mortality of hospitalized children (Eppich, Adler, & McGaghie, 2006; Sam, Pierse, Al-Qahtani, & Cheng, 2012). To adequately prepare clinicians to treat these rare but acute conditions, which carry a heavy burden of potential morbidity, is a constant challenge that it is perilous to neglect. Compounding that challenge, newer medications and advances in technology enable many patients to survive high-acuity disease states that in the past were fatal.

Medical personnel who train in pediatrics face a dearth of opportunities to develop their assessment and acute care skills. Opportunities to treat emergencies are highly limited so that, as Cheng and colleagues noted, many of the relevant skills "are taught didactically, with few opportunities for hands-on practice" (Cheng, Duff, Grant, Kissoon, & Grant, 2007, p. 466). Just because severe respiratory failure is an infrequent but high-risk event, care is likely to be heavily supervised and conducted by senior staff, limiting the exposure and decision-making autonomy of trainees. Restrictions on work hours; increasing emphasis on outpatient pediatrics; and the high-risk, low-frequency nature of acute care events all limit opportunities to learn in clinical situations. However, at the same time, the need for providers with such emergency skills is growing because more children survive congenital syndromes and significant prematurity. Many of these children are also technology-dependent for survival and their resuscitation during acute illness requires a unique set of technical and assessment skills.

As in other specialties, however, simulation in pediatrics is relatively novel for most clinicians. Recognition, at least from academic sources, that pediatricians were insufficiently trained in resuscitation is not new (Nadel et al., 2000). But for most members on pediatric teams who trained for the specialty prior to 2000, simulation was not a part of their educational experience, either for learning or for assessment.

SIMULATION AND THE INTERPROFESSIONAL IMPERATIVE

By the time that *To Err Is Human* was first published at the turn of the 21st century, academic pediatricians had already evinced concern about reported deficiencies in resuscitation and life-saving skills among residents (Maibach, Schieber, & Carroll, 1996; Nadel et al., 2000; White, Shugerman, Brownlee, & Quan, 1998). Initiating a program in neonatal resuscitation, Halamek and colleagues called for a "new paradigm" in pediatrics education as early as 2000 (Halamek et al., 2000). Five years later, Weinstock and colleagues at Harvard Medical School described their installation of a simulation suite in a tertiary care hospital (Weinstock et al., 2005). Other publications percolated through the pediatric literature through the first decade of the century. In 2007 Cheng described simulation in pediatrics as "an educational revolution" and pointed to its basis in experiential and reflective learning (Cheng et al., 2007). The next year saw the first meeting of the International Pediatric Simulation Symposia and Workshops (International Pediatric Simulation Society).

Emphasis on interprofessional learning has grown together with interest in simulation in pediatrics (van Schaik, Plant, Diane, Tsang, & O'Sullivan, 2011). A single individual is unlikely to possess the requisite knowledge base to properly assess, decide upon, and undertake the optimal treatment. Consequently, to avoid mistakes and provide the best care, it is crucial that teams function seamlessly. Their composition may include physician specialists, the primary bedside physician, bedside nurses, advanced practice nurses, physician assistants, respiratory therapists, clinical educators, and administrative staff.

Cohen's Children's Medical Center is a tertiary care hospital that includes quaternary care surgical and medical programs; it is the largest provider of pediatric services in New York State and includes neonatal facilities and an extensive emergency service that receives more than 37,000 patients annually. Consequently, we have developed a broad-based series of simulation programs with a view to continuous quality improvement in acute care contexts for instances of sudden life-threatening emergencies. The overall aim is to enhance interprofessional communication and teamwork, systems evaluation and patient safety, and also to discover latent safety threats. Other programs include initiatives for clinical teams to manage common conditions and efforts to improve communications during stressful interactions (see Chapter 9).

Of the three programs described in this chapter, all contend with aspects of emergency care. Each is targeted to specific interprofessional teams that form in the context of acute care, including transport teams and teams created on the spot to attend to sudden emergencies on the hospital floor. We craft scenarios for high-fidelity, manikin-based simulations and include standardized patients as confederates. Two of our programs run scenarios at the Patient Safety Institute (PSI); the third is an in-situ program that takes place at various locations in the hospital—distinctive in that it is unannounced to staff beforehand.

Pediatric Acute Care Assessment, Stabilization, and Escalation (PASS)

The vast majority of pediatric inpatient resuscitations involve progressive respiratory insufficiency leading to acute respiratory failure or hemodynamic compromise. Timely recognition of subtle signs and symptoms before significant morbidity occurs should be the primary goal of any inpatient safety initiative. Our PASS program targets pediatric resident trainees and floor nursing staff because they are most often the identifiers of, and primary responders to, these conditions, responsible for the early recognition of decompensating patients. Typically, three or four resident physicians and two or three nurses join us for a series of three to four scenarios. Our scenarios include learning objectives that are both general, related to appropriate behavior at all stages of patient care, and specific with respect to the condition being simulated.

Case History: Sepsis in a 6-Year-Old Child[1] An emergency in which time to recognition and treatment are crucial components, sepsis can arise from what appear to be benign injuries; untreated or undertreated, it can readily lead to septic shock with severe risk of mortality (Parker, 2009). We run a hybrid simulation with a high-fidelity manikin and one standardized patient who portrays a parent, generally the mother. The scenario is broken down into three phases and lasts approximately 20 minutes, to be followed by a full debriefing that may last as long as an hour. The action takes place in an emergency bay at PSI, with remote observation of participants and "on-the-fly" vocalization of the computerized manikin.

Triage History The patient is a 6-year-old male, Ben Fletcher; his mother, Alice, provides the history. For 3 days, Ben has suffered high fever. "He's been running a temperature of 103°F." He has vomited repeatedly and complained of abdominal pain. Just yesterday he saw a pediatrician, who diagnosed gastrointestinal disease and prescribed Zofran. But because he continued to feel sick, Alice brought him to the emergency department (ED).

Phase I (0 to 5 Minutes) As she replies to the questions participants ask, Alice is visibly upset and anxious. The child has no allergies and takes no medications; he has no past medical history. He last ate at 8:00 that morning but can't keep anything down; he continues to vomit. He last voided urine yesterday. To Alice, Ben appears gray and sickly.

"I feel like I'm going to throw up," Ben himself says. "My belly hurts."

His temperature is indeed elevated at 40.1°C and on examination his lips and mouth are dry and cracked. His heart rate trends upward from 130 (sinus) to 150 beats per minute (bpm) over the course of a few minutes, while his blood pressure drops to 70/50. Circulation shows a gallop rhythm with a soft holosystolic murmur, 2+ pulses, and a capillary refill of 4 seconds. When his abdomen is touched, he screams in pain.

Observers note, as they watch the simulation play out from a remote booth during this first phase, whether participants engage in a series of crucial tasks in addition to obtaining a rapid history. They should assign team roles, ensure an open airway, and administer immediate supplemental oxygen. With intravenous insertion there should come a request for a rapid infuser for a fluid bolus. In addition to initiating continuous monitoring, the team should order chest and abdominal x-rays and a complete blood workup. The proper airway equipment called for should include a bag-valve mask, nonrebreather mask, and endotracheal tube suction. The team should request ceftriaxone for intraosseous infusion and note that metabolic derangement in sepsis requires treatment with blood glucose.

Phase II (6 to 15 Minutes) Ben's mother grows increasingly and visibly upset as we move into the second phase of the scenario. Alice insistently asks, "How sick is my Ben? Will he get better? He's going to get better, isn't he? How long is this going to take? Can you tell me how this happened? I thought he had the stomach flu." Like many parents in an acute situation at a teaching hospital, Alice evinces fear that something is going wrong but that the providers will not tell her what it is. "Are you doing research on my child? Is this an experiment? Don't you know what's wrong?"

Meanwhile, Ben's heart rate continues to increase to 180 bpm while his blood pressure continues to drop as low as 70/30. The team should both treat the patient with pain medication and provide sedation while making the key observation, as indicated by monitoring, that Ben is not improving with administration of fluids; he continues to be in shock. This should alert the team that rapid sequence induction is called for, to be performed with cricoid pressure for intubation. The team should also request a postintubation chest x-ray, which the observers provide. Because Ben does not improve with administration of fluids, the team should request vasopressor infusion.

Phase III (16 to 20 Minutes) Vasopressor administration brings about rapid improvement of blood pressure and heart rate returns to high normal range over the course of 3 minutes.

Extensive Debrief For this case, we focus on the first steps and critical early maneuvers in assessing and treating this patient. Rather than emphasizing the algorithms associated with pediatric advanced life support (PALS) in clinical situations that require higher levels of expertise and training, we ensure that participants understand the basis for, and can effectively deploy, the crucial first steps, such as the head-tilt-chin lift. Under stress of circumstance, which includes the external pressure from the patient's mother, team members may experience difficulty with bag-valve mask ventilation, a procedure that should be performed in a controlled and systematic fashion. Typically, there is a tendency with airway-related cases for trainees to move beyond basic procedures and attempt advanced interventions, such as rapid endotracheal intubation, that they normally would not perform without supervision.

Critical Care–Emergent Stabilization and Transport Program

Our medical center is responsible for transporting critically ill children throughout our catchment area, which includes all of Long Island and three of New York City's five boroughs: Queens, Brooklyn, and Staten Island. Our critical care nurses both triage and conduct over 3,800 neonatal and pediatric critical care transports yearly. Some cases require, due to the level of illness of the patient, that a critical care physician-in-training accompany the team. Initial assessment, stabilization, and transport of these patients often require complex clinical decisions and the execution of challenging procedures in less-than-ideal environments under stressful conditions.

Case History: Tension Pneumothorax in a 12-Year-Old Pedestrian Struck by a Vehicle Transporting a patient from an ED to an intensive care unit (ICU) can invoke a range of medical issues as well as conflictual interactions among emergency and transport personnel, complicated by extreme distress on the part of a parent. Information received from the referring party requesting transport determines the decision as to team composition. Our teams include an experienced ICU or best practice nurse, or a nurse practitioner, and, as in the case we recount here, may include a pulmonary specialist. For these hybrid scenarios we employ confederates who portray an attending physician, a nurse in the ED and, in addition, an anxious and upset parent. We build a variety of components into the extemporaneous play of the scenario, which, as happens frequently in transfer situations, obstruct optimal assessment and decision making on the part of the transport team.

Phase I (0 to 5 Minutes) Information the team receives for this case prior to their arrival at the ED is minimal. The patient (manikin), Brianna Carter, is a 12-year-old girl who was struck by an automobile. Unconscious when emergency personnel arrive, the team learns that she was intubated at the scene of the accident; however, en route to the ED, she regained consciousness and extubated herself, a potentially life-threatening complication. The attending physician reintubated and initiated mild sedation. He or she recognized that the patient required intensive care and called for transport.

Entering the ED, the team finds Brianna to be semiconscious, moaning, but unable to make coherent responses to questions. Her vital signs indicate distress, with a heart rate of 140 bpm and blood pressure 90/50; her respiratory rate is 22 breaths per minute with SaO2 91%. Most significantly, auscultation indicates no breath sounds on the right side.

Observers pay specific attention, during this initial phase of the scenario, to the transport nurses' and physician's overall assessment and stabilization efforts within their scope of practice. First actions should include, with respect to the child's rapid respiration, confirmation of tube placement and assurance that it is fully advanced into the trachea. The team should also determine that proper sedation has been administered, both in terms of medication and dosage.

The interactive component of the scenario creates challenges from the outset. Brianna's mother is anxious to have the transport team rush the child to the hospital, but, by contrast, the physician evinces defensive annoyance. Comments from the emergency physician include:

"The kid has some trauma but is okay. . . . Of course we intubated. . . . You can see that. . . . We need an ambulance, not a platoon. I'm only following protocol. You guys are just pediatricians. Scared of everything."

The team thus finds itself in a typical bind and must respond to a series of challenges related to professionalism. On one hand the physician has called for transport; at the same time, he or she feels territorially encroached upon by the team and, as a matter of psychological defense, makes aggressive suggestions and may react unpleasantly if he feels threatened. In transport simulation, frequent behavior of this kind warrants the use of an obstreperous confederate.

Phase II (5 to 10 Minutes) Vital signs tend toward an indication of advanced distress as blood pressure drops to 70/45 and respiration rate rises to 30, with heart rate spikes and premature ventricular contractions (PVCs)—another sign the significance of which the attending physician will contest.

Teams vary in their response at this point in the scenario. Some will immediately apply a bag-valve mask and recognize that the patient requires needle decompression of the right chest. If they take these steps to improve oxygen saturation and attend to the pneumothorax, the patient's vital signs will rapidly return to normal. If not, the patient will continue to deteriorate, with the heart rate rising to 170 bpm and several PVCs each minute; blood pressure will continue downward with diastolic to 40 and respiration will rise to 35. At all events, the team should be reporting their findings to base.

Phase III (10 to 15 Minutes) If the team fails to recognize the urgent requirement for needle decompression, the patient will progress toward cardiac arrest with pulseless electrical activity (PEA). Without attention to the pneumothorax, there is no return to normal circulation.

Extensive Debrief Both clinical and organizational components come under discussion in debriefs for transport scenarios. Assessment, stabilization and/or management, and the decision to escalate are the key components, while the ability to assemble the team, designate roles, and open lines of communication are crucial for clinical performance. We emphasize the fundamentals and stepwise approach to treating pneumothorax—first ensuring that the endotracheal tube is in the right position, for example, and that IV access is good.

Team members' situational awareness and self-awareness also constitute important boundaries for the actions they take and, based on the participants' level of training, we emphasize these core elements during debriefs. A pediatric resident should beware, for example, of administering sedative medication to an acutely ill patient if he or she has yet to learn to perform skilled airway management. An ICU fellow might not be prepared to do needle decompression, and even an attending physician may be confronted with an emergency situation that warrants restraint before action: when, for example, a head trauma injury calls for surgery that would be appropriate only with recourse to a neurosurgeon or some degree of supervision or backup. We make every effort in transport scenarios to instill in learners the importance of building a mental model that includes awareness of the limits to their skills and their scope of practice. A mainstay of the educational focus in debriefing is to help participants identify a reasonable framework for safe and timely escalation.

In-Situ Simulation Program

The hospital itself, understood as comprised of multiple environments within a complex infrastructure and complicated design matrix, includes any number of ready-made "sets" for in-situ simulation scenarios. Although nurses, physicians, and other staff are in principle trained to follow protocols to contend with the various infrequent pediatric emergencies, these sudden events may occur anywhere within the hospital at any time. Simulation can reveal serious hazards and latent environmental threats posed by equipment and supplies and their ready availability. It can point to issues in interdependence between departments, discrepancies in policies, and, more generally, problems with the culture of the organization (Rosen, Hunt, Pronovost, Federowicz, & Weaver, 2012). Particularly egregious threats may be observed in services that pediatrics generally share with adult facilities, such as radiology, in which personnel may be wholly unprepared for emergencies with young patients.

Novel Aims, Multiple Uses

In the pediatrics literature, reports on in-situ simulation show that it has been utilized in diverse ways in various health systems, both as a pedagogical tool as well as an evolving method to survey systems and human factors. Latent safety threats constitute one focus of the in-situ approach. Performing 64 in-situ simulations over the course of 21 months, Wheeler and colleagues noted more than 134 latent safety threats and knowledge gaps in areas such as medication, equipment, and resources/care delivery systems; their identification resulted in implementation of policies, education, and resources to enhance the safety culture of their system (Wheeler, Geis, Mack, Lemaster, & Patterson, 2013). In obstetrics, particularly, several teams have reported introduction of mobile in-situ obstetrics emergency simulation as an effective and well-received way to reduce latent threats (Guise et al., 2010; Hamman et al., 2009; Hamman et al., 2010). A group in New Zealand reported consistent latent errors related to introduction of new resuscitation equipment (Garden et al., 2010).

Studies of in-situ simulation have also reported success with response times and appropriate escalation. One group reported that its in-situ multidisciplinary teamwork training program improved mean overall ER resuscitation time by 16% and, as well, substantially better near-perfect task completion (Steinemann et al., 2011). Regular in-situ training of a pediatric medical emergency response team resulted in earlier recognition of critical illness, and higher levels of appropriate escalation of care that then extended to a reduction in PICU length of stay and mortality (Theilen et al., 2013).

Finally, health care unit design has become a growing challenge. New technologies add layers of complexity; so, too, does the necessity to reorient personnel toward a team-based interdisciplinary approach and the need for heightened situational awareness, fewer distractions, and task fixation. Several recent reports on in-situ simulation address macrosystems configuration. Patterson and colleagues have been pioneers in efforts to investigate system–human interaction factors and latent safety threats prior to start up, using the lessons they learned to inform the design of a pediatric ER (Patterson, Geis, Falcone, LeMaster, & Wears, 2013). One group has described what it learned from a community hospital-wide fire simulation (Hohenhaus et al., 2008). In a high-risk obstetrics service, in-situ simulation was used to identify defensive barriers and classify active and latent breaches (Riley, Davis, Miller, Hansen, & Sweet, 2010). In brief, a broad-based systems approach using in-situ simulation can help identify gaps, redundancies, and commonly breached protective layers in safety systems.

Preserving Situational Fidelity With No Prior Announcement Our in-situ program is distinctive in that we run simulations *unannounced* within various units and at different locations in the hospital. In developing this model, with its focus on delivery of acute care to manage rare events, we enlisted the support of the hospital administration and alerted in writing and in meetings with the nursing and physician leadership. Personnel on units, floors, and in all relevant locations were informed that simulations would take place without prior announcement, noting that none of the information gathered would be attributed to individuals, inserted into employee records, or used for retribution.

In-situ simulations may adapt any of the emergency scenarios concerned with respiratory, cardiac, or accident-related emergencies. We generally use trained confederates in addition to high-fidelity manikins and adopt the three-phase model, as in our PASS and transport programs. We deploy to the main pavilions and units, including such service areas as the emergency bay, pediatric

ICU, trauma unit, or radiology suite. Our aims are several, including team formation and response, identification of issues in assessment and management, and also—unique to the in-situ format—potential threats related to hospital infrastructure and design, handoff, equipment readiness, supplies availability, and interdepartmental flow and systems processes.

Contending With Resistance In spite of providing blanket information that in-situ simulations will take place unannounced, pushback and resistance on the part of staff are common and to be expected. Nurse managers and nurses will resist the sudden imposition of a scenario and comments such as, "We're really busy," and, "I can't believe you want to start this sort of thing right now," are common. Pointing out that emergencies occur during busy periods is a reasonable response; they may also occur when a floor is "understaffed." In our experience, resistance on any given unit waxes and wanes; it is greater at night than during the day.

Prebriefing/Introduction We state aloud the basic assumption that we bring to in-situ simulation. "We believe that, as a participant, each of you is intelligent, well-trained, want to do your best, and to improve your performance. This is an opportunity to practice patient care, teamwork, and communication in a safe and supportive environment, using simulation. The manikin and personnel who simulate the patient or the patient's family members have limitations. Please do your best to suspend disbelief and act as you would with a real patient and family."

Crew Resource Management (CRM)/Teamwork Response The actual number of participants at any given location varies widely, from three to four to upwards from 15 to 20. Part of the exercise involves the leader assembling the team and excluding unneeded personnel. We may also note the challenges that teams face in identifying a leader. During the course of the scenario they may provide inconsistent or incomplete information during handoff to the ICU. They may be challenged with respect to situational awareness or fail, for example, to request a handoff when one is called for. They may have difficulty with closed-loop communications and in identifying or developing the appropriate mental model and sharing it with the team.

Issues in Assessment/Resuscitation/Stabilization Specific performance gaps have been the hallmark of our in-situ simulations that involve this fundamental set of low-frequency events. Among them we could include application of the bag-valve mask without the head-tilt jaw thrust; failure to use a backboard with cardiopulmonary resuscitation (CPR); administration of epinephrine before observation of anaphylactic shock; and failure to recognize ventricular tachycardia. Any number of such gaps may be related to failures of assessment and unfamiliarity with code procedures.

Some performance gaps are due to the fact that the simulation occurs in an area of the hospital typically shared by pediatrics with adult services. Personnel in nuclear medicine, for example, rarely see pediatric patients and the unit itself is not equipped for resuscitation. These circumstances can also lead to delay in recognizing emergencies.

Other typical performance gaps include telecommunications errors, such as calling in the wrong code type or failure to specify a location. As in all emergency pediatric simulations, we also identify instances of interventions outside the provider's scope of practice.

Equipment and Infrastructure Issues that in day-to-day practice in a hospital pose no particular problem can constitute serious latent safety threats during an emergency. Lack of code documentation sheets on a code cart, for example, may entail serious confusion in handoff of the patient to the ICU staff. Low battery charge or difficulties in attaching the defibrillator to the pad system are just two examples of equipment-related failures that can cost time, and sometimes lives, in emergencies. Less-than-ideal positioning of equipment, such as bag-valve masks, or lack of age-appropriate size masks, can delay rescue breathing and result in a hypoxic patient developing further distress or cardiac arrest. Misplaced medications in the resuscitation cart can add to confusion during an acute emergency and contribute to either dosing or wrong-drug errors.

Value of Targeted Programs

Pediatric health care providers must capably and skillfully contend with life-threatening emergencies that afflict young patients who more often than not have limited abilities to communicate verbally. The very infrequency of these events and the specific procedures required to address them, together with parents' anxiety, are all complicating features that favor learning through simulation. Crafting scenarios that address these issues in a variety of environments, together with provision for extensive debriefing, provides individuals and interprofessional teams with the tools and means to deliberately practice both hands-on and communications skills. They offer occasions to organize and improve skill sets, enhance scientific and applied knowledge, and raise situational awareness during emergencies and other high-risk events; they can also reveal latent safety threats.

NOTE

1. Case developed in collaboration with Linda L. Brown, MD (Hasbro Children's Hospital, Brown University).

REFERENCES

Cheng, A., Duff, J., Grant, E., Kissoon, N., & Grant, V. J. (2007). Simulation in paediatrics: An educational revolution. *Paediatrics and Child Health, 12*(6), 465–468.

Eppich, W. J., Adler, M. D., & McGaghie, W. C. (2006). Emergency and critical care pediatrics: Use of medical simulation for training in acute pediatric emergencies. *Current Opinion in Pediatrics, 18*(3), 266–271. doi:10.1097/01.mop.0000193309.22462.c9

Garden, A. L., Mills, S. A., Wilson, R., Watts, P., Griffin, J. M., Gannon, S., & Kapoor, I. (2010). In situ simulation training for paediatric cardiorespiratory arrest: Initial observations and identification of latent errors. *Anaesthesia and Intensive Care, 38*(6), 1038–1042.

Guise, J. M., Lowe, N. K., Deering, S., Lewis, P. O., O'Haire, C., Irwin, L. K., . . . Kanki, B. G. (2010). Mobile in situ obstetric emergency simulation and teamwork training to improve maternal-fetal safety in hospitals. *Joint Commission Journal on Quality and Patient Safety, 36*(10), 443–453.

Halamek, L. P., Kaegi, D. M., Gaba, D. M., Sowb, Y. A., Smith, B. C., Smith, B. E., & Howard, S. K. (2000). Time for a new paradigm in pediatric medical education: Teaching neonatal resuscitation in a simulated delivery room environment. *Pediatrics, 106*(4), E45.

Hamman, W. R., Beaudin-Seiler, B. M., Beaubien, J. M., Gullickson, A. M., Gross, A. C., Orizondo-Korotko, K., . . . Lammers, R. (2009). Using in situ simulation to identify and resolve latent environmental threats to patient safety: Case study involving a labor and delivery ward. *Journal of Patient Safety, 5*(3), 184–187. doi:10.1097/PTS.0b013e3181b35e6c

Hamman, W. R., Beaudin-Seiler, B. M., Beaubien, J. M., Gullickson, A. M., Orizondo-Korotko, K., Gross, A. C., . . . Lammers, R. (2010). Using in situ simulation to identify and resolve latent environmental threats to patient safety: Case study involving operational changes in a labor and delivery ward. *Quality Management in Health Care, 19*(3), 226–230. doi:10.1097/QMH. 0b013e3181eb1452

Hohenhaus, S. M., Hohenhaus, J., Saunders, M., Vandergrift, J., Kohler, T. A., Manikowski, M. E., . . . Holleran, S. (2008). Emergency response: Lessons learned during a community hospital's in situ fire simulation. *Journal of Emergency Nursing, 34*(4), 352–354. doi:10.1016/j. jen.2008.04.025

International Pediatric Simulation Society. Retrieved from http://www.ipedsim.com/gathermeetings/ aboutipssw

Maibach, E. W., Schieber, R. A., & Carroll, M. F. (1996). Self-efficacy in pediatric resuscitation: Implications for education and performance. *Pediatrics, 97*(1), 94–99.

Nadel, F. M., Lavelle, J. M., Fein, J. A., Giardino, A. P., Decker, J. M., & Durbin, D. R. (2000). Assessing pediatric senior residents' training in resuscitation: Fund of knowledge, technical skills, and perception of confidence. *Pediatric Emergency Care, 16*(2), 73–76.

Parker, M. M. (2009). Pediatric sepsis: Time is of the essence. *Critical Care Medicine, 37*(2), 785–786. doi:10.1097/CCM.0b013e3181931210

Patterson, M. D., Geis, G. L., Falcone, R. A., LeMaster, T., & Wears, R. L. (2013). In situ simulation: Detection of safety threats and teamwork training in a high risk emergency department. *BMJ Quality and Safety, 22*(6), 468–477. doi:10.1136/bmjqs-2012-000942

Riley, W., Davis, S., Miller, K. M., Hansen, H., & Sweet, R. M. (2010). Detecting breaches in defensive barriers using in situ simulation for obstetric emergencies. *Quality and Safety in Health Care, 19*(Suppl. 3), i53–i56. doi:10.1136/qshc.2010.040311

Rosen, M. A., Hunt, E. A., Pronovost, P. J., Federowicz, M. A., & Weaver, S. J. (2012). In situ simulation in continuing education for the health care professions: A systematic review. *The Journal of Continuing Education in the Health Professions, 32*(4), 243–254. doi:10.1002/ chp.21152

Sam, J., Pierse, M., Al-Qahtani, A., & Cheng, A. (2012). Implementation and evaluation of a simulation curriculum for paediatric residency programs including just-in-time in situ mock codes. *Paediatrics and Child Health, 17*(2), e16–e20.

Steinemann, S., Berg, B., Skinner, A., DiTulio, A., Anzelon, K., Terada, K., . . . Speck, C. (2011). In situ, multidisciplinary, simulation-based teamwork training improves early trauma care. *Journal of Surgical Education, 68*(6), 472–477. doi:10.1016/j.jsurg.2011.05.009

Theilen, U., Leonard, P., Jones, P., Ardill, R., Weitz, J., Agrawal, D., & Simpson, D. (2013). Regular in situ simulation training of paediatric medical emergency team improves hospital response to deteriorating patients. *Resuscitation, 84*(2), 218–222. doi:10.1016/j. resuscitation.2012.06.027

van Schaik, S. M., Plant, J., Diane, S., Tsang, L., & O'Sullivan, P. (2011). Interprofessional team training in pediatric resuscitation: A low-cost, in situ simulation program that enhances self-efficacy among participants. *Clinical Pediatrics (Phila), 50*(9), 807–815. doi:10.1177/0009922811405518

Weinstock, P. H., Kappus, L. J., Kleinman, M. E., Grenier, B., Hickey, P., & Burns, J. P. (2005). Toward a new paradigm in hospital-based pediatric education: The development of an onsite simulator program. *Pediatric Critical Care Medicine, 6*(6), 635–641.

Wheeler, D. S., Geis, G., Mack, E. H., Lemaster, T., & Patterson, M. D. (2013). High-reliability emergency response teams in the hospital: Improving quality and safety using in situ simulation training. *BMJ Quality and Safety, 22*(6), 507–514. doi:10.1136/bmjqs-2012-000931

White, J. R., Shugerman, R., Brownlee, C., & Quan, L. (1998). Performance of advanced resuscitation skills by pediatric housestaff. *Archives of Pediatrics and Adolescent Medicine, 152*(12), 1232–1235.

Helen Maliagros Scott
John Perrone
Andrew Drozd

9: Dimensions in Pediatrics Simulation: Teamwork and Communication

Simulation in pediatrics is not limited to use with rare and acute conditions, but extends to the everyday challenges often encountered in providing care to young patients. An interprofessional simulation program introduces junior pediatric residents and novice nurses to common conditions seen in the hospital setting, with scenarios designed to augment diagnostic and management skills, to enhance teamwork and communications, and to ensure teams are prepared to take appropriate steps in escalation of care. For senior residents, in addition, simulation targets some of their most difficult interactions with patients and family members, including delivery of bad news, admitting a mistake, suspicion of child abuse, and other issues with acute emotional components. Plans to evaluate these programs include the use of multisource feedback.

Challenges confront pediatrics educators today in terms of providing high-quality learning opportunities and optimal exposure to a wide variety of conditions. Concern for patient safety frequently makes it difficult if not impossible to teach, as in the past, in the immediate context of clinical practice. The old model of "see one, do one, teach one" is anachronistic while the infrequency of most pediatric medical emergencies provides trainees with few opportunities for hands-on learning (Yager, Lok, & Klig, 2011). In addition, treating children, even under the best of circumstances, involves recognition of behavioral and developmental nuances and the sorts of demanding social interactions that, for

the novice learner, can prove stressful. "[O]ne may argue that the ethical imperative for simulation is stronger in pediatrics than in any other field of health care"
(Halamek & Yaeger, 2008, p. 338).

For all these reasons, simulation in interprofessional contexts has proven to
be an invaluable supplement to the education and postgraduate training of registered nurses, residents, and other health care providers. Basic "mock code" programs that use simple manikins or task trainers are insufficiently realistic and
generally do not include facilitated debriefing (Grant, Duff, Bhanji, & Cheng,
2013). However, simulation that improves teamwork, defined as "those behaviors that facilitate effective interaction" (Beaubien & Baker, 2004, p. i51), allows
participants to practice, in a safe environment, leadership skills and mutual performance monitoring, as well as clinical decision-making and task-related skills
(van Schaik, Plant, Diane, Tsang, & O'Sullivan, 2011). To be effective, simulation also requires structured feedback through the debrief process; active participation; and appropriate environmental, psychological, and physical fidelity
(Issenberg, McGaghie, Petrusa, Lee Gordon, & Scalese, 2005).

An Interprofessional Clinical Teams Program

We use high-fidelity simulation and scenarios with standardized patients to
familiarize first-year pediatric residents and recently graduated nurses with some
of the common illnesses seen in hospitalized patients. Our program aims both to
instruct learners and to improve team dynamics in the inpatient setting. In addition
to the diminishing opportunities for clinical practice accorded trainees as noted
in the preceding, we have also been motivated by work-hour restrictions and by
enhanced supervision required of attending physicians—both owing to increasing patient safety concerns (Oshimura, Sperring, Bauer, & Rauch, 2012; Peets &
Ayas, 2012).

Goals and Objectives Clinical conditions chosen for our interprofessional
pediatrics simulation-based courses are those the faculty consider common
occurrences in a hospital setting and which may require rapid intervention to
avoid patient decompensation. We have developed scenarios for such conditions as status asthmaticus, neonatal sepsis, status epilepticus, anaphylaxis, and
bronchiolitis, among others.

Organization and Play of the Scenario We give the course on a monthly
basis to groups that include three to five pediatric residents and one to three
pediatric medical–surgical nurses. Each course takes place at the Patient Safety
Institute (PSI) and lasts approximately 4 hours. Faculty members, who observe
the scenarios and facilitate the subsequent debriefs, generally include a pediatric attending physician from the Department of Hospital Medicine, one or two
clinical education specialists from PSI, and a nurse educator.

To initiate a scenario, we present the goals and specific objectives of the
course and explain that, in addition to gaining experience and confidence in
detecting and managing common pediatric conditions, including appropriate
escalation of care, the overall aim is to improve teamwork and communication among the first-line staff in a hospital setting. In terms of clinical goals,

at the end of this course, participants are expected to have shown that they are able to take an accurate history and perform an appropriate physical exam on a pediatric patient, identify and manage common childhood conditions in the hospital setting, know when and how to escalate care, and demonstrate awareness of the possible complications of each condition. They should also be able to effectively communicate and interact with the patient, family members, other team members, and to demonstrate an understanding of the roles that other disciplines play in treating each condition under consideration.

The basic team for each simulation consists of a resident and pediatric nurse; ancillary personnel may also participate. To the group we read a short introduction that provides the patient's name, age, weight, pertinent history, and any interventions prior to the clinical encounter. Nonparticipant members of the group observe the scenario unfold on video monitor; each scenario is videotaped and can be played back as needed during the subsequent debriefing. Each resident and nurse participates in at least one clinical scenario during the session.

Finally, each scenario has its own set of learning objectives; these are reviewed and discussed at the end of the debrief session. During this time, the clinical "pearls"—instances of condensed clinically relevant information—of each case are reviewed (Lorin, Palazzi, Turner, & Ward, 2008). There is no formal, written evaluation of the participants, so as to make the course as nonthreatening as possible.

Interprofessional Teams Clinical Example: Anaphylaxis

The setting for this scenario is the pediatric medical–surgical unit. We read the introduction aloud:

> Mary is a 2-year-old female with no significant past medical history. She has been admitted to the medical–surgical unit for dehydration secondary to acute gastroenteritis. She is doing well and will be discharged after lunch, which she is eating now. Halfway through lunch, however, Mary's mother comes to tell you that Mary has broken out into a rash and bumps all over her body. When you walk into the room, you will find the patient with a diffuse urticarial rash that appears to be pruritic; her lips and eyes are swollen.

When the participants enter, they find the patient in respiratory distress. She has hives and swelling, and upon auscultation she also wheezes diffusely while retracting subcostally. She is tachypneic at 30 breaths per minute. Oxygen saturation remains 93% to 95%. She is afebrile and slightly tachycardic to 120 beats per minute. Blood pressure is stable at 90/50. She is crying and anxious and will not answer questions.

Mrs. Gwynn, Mary's mother—a standardized patient/confederate—is extremely nervous and upset. Nothing like this has ever happened to her child and she doesn't understand what could be wrong. She is frustrated because she was told Mary would be discharged today. She blames the hospital: there must have been something wrong with the food. Mrs. Gwynn is emotionally wrought, sobbing, and concerned that Mary's rash, swelling, and breathing are worsening rapidly.

Observation to Assess Objectives

Faculty, both instructors and facilitators, observe the scenario as it plays out and note whether team members acquire the information they need through focused questioning and timely recognition that the patient's symptoms indicate a diagnosis of anaphylaxis (Table 9.1). They watch to see whether the team formulates a management plan and properly administers epinephrine, and how they interact with the patient and parent, both in terms of the quality of information they provide and their interpersonal skills in contending with a child in crisis and a mother in distress.

Extensive Debrief Facilitators include the attending physician, the nurse educator, and clinical education specialists. When scenarios include confederates or standardized patients, we request they stay in character and share their impressions of the participants' professionalism, teamwork, clinical skills, and ability to communicate. Observers share their thoughts and experiences with similar situations, and give recommendations; the group discusses the type and quality of team interaction between resident and nurse.

Communication and Professionalism Program

As a result of its influential Outcome Project, implemented from 2002 to 2008, the Accreditation Council for Graduate Medical Education (ACGME) identifies six core competencies as requisite in residency training (Ling, Derstine, & Cohen, 2013). Interpersonal and communication skills as well as professionalism constitute two of these six (Table 9.2), integral to physician development.

TABLE 9.1 Observing Team Members and Assessing Teamwork

Data Gathering	To be able to ask focused questions in an emergent situation
	To quickly assess and share appropriate vital signs and physical findings with the team
Recognition	To rapidly identify a clinical emergency
	To recognize signs and symptoms of anaphylaxis
	To recognize abnormal vital signs
Management	To know the critical steps needed to treat anaphylaxis and to administer epinephrine rapidly and appropriately
	To understand the treatment (acute and long term) of an anaphylactic reaction
	To anticipate the possible complications of anaphylaxis and its interventions
	To effectively communicate diagnosis, treatment, and ongoing management to family members
Teamwork	To effectively communicate findings and the plan of care to all team members and delegate tasks in an efficient and appropriate manner

TABLE 9.2 Accreditation Council for Graduate Medical Education (ACGME) Six Core Competencies

1. Medical knowledge
2. Patient care
3. Professionalism
4. Interpersonal communication
5. Practice-based learning: personal improvement
6. System-based practice: system improvement

The ACGME states that interpersonal and communication skills "result in effective information exchange and teaming with patients, their families, and other health professionals" and professionalism "as manifested through a commitment to carrying out professional responsibilities, adherence to ethical principles, and sensitivity to a diverse patient population" (cited in Brinkman et al., 2006, p. 1372).

In general, professionalism and effective communication skills have been shown to successfully increase patient satisfaction, understanding, and compliance, with proficiency in these competencies linked to improved clinical outcomes (Issenberg, Chung, & Devine, 2011; Swing, 2007). However, teaching these skills to residents can be challenging. While the other ACGME core competencies, such as medical knowledge and systems-based learning, can be taught using more conventional methods such as lectures, didactics, and reading assignments, skills such as professionalism and communication are not so readily acquired. They are highly individualized, cultivated over many years, and not easily quantified. For these reasons, education in communication and professionalism requires more guidance, practice, and experiential learning.

The ability to communicate effectively takes on special importance for pediatricians, who treat children of all ages and sizes, most often with highly limited understanding or the ability to express themselves verbally. In addition, while communication with young patients requires finesse and knowledge of age-appropriate language, it is often the family, usually distraught and in crisis, that proves the most challenging to interact with.

Communications Challenges: Four Cases

Our communication and professionalism program essentially targets advanced residents. We have developed a library of scenarios, most of which were inspired and shaped by actual cases that occurred in various units of our pediatric tertiary-care hospital. Frequently, these concern situations that had escalated and were referred to senior leadership in the hospital, or which led to medical errors or near misses owing to lapses in communication. In the following, we summarize four of these scenarios, together with directions provided to the standardized patients who take the role of parent or other family member.

Our decision to use actual cases that occurred in our health system as the basis for simulation scenarios, instead of developing case material from written sources or based on schematic principles, offered several advantages. In particular, we could make use of the high degree of cultural diversity found within our catchment area in ways that highlight issues of genuine concern to our residents and teams. Subjects and topics among our scenarios include parents who use herbs and teas in place of insulin for their diabetic child, adolescents struggling with sexual identity, South Asian parental distrust of Western medicine, and Jehovah's Witnesses and the problem of blood transfusion.

In addition to drawing upon the cultural conflicts and values actually encountered in our health system, the use of real source material has the additional advantage of turning to good use institutional or organizational memory, as we describe more fully in the following, and also with respect to developing reliable evaluations of residents in ways that can meet ACGME standards.

Case 1: Admitting a Mistake John is a 10-month-old infant who was admitted to your unit—*we explain to the resident*—with hyponatremic dehydration secondary to vomiting and diarrhea. Initially his sodium level was 125 and currently, 12 hours after admission, it is 128. You have been monitoring electrolytes by blood draws once every 4 hours since initiation of treatment in the emergency department and adjusting IV fluids accordingly. John's parents are becoming increasingly alarmed, frustrated, and upset. Each blood draw requires multiple attempts by residents, attending physicians, and nurses. His parents do not understand the necessity to take blood so often, especially because he is so tired and ill.

This morning, after a similar ordeal, you finally obtained a blood specimen for a basic metabolic panel. You immediately sent it to the laboratory to be processed. Twenty minutes later, you receive a call from the laboratory director, who tells you that the specimen arrived without a label and therefore cannot be processed. You do not remember placing a label on the tube before you sent it to the lab. After several minutes of pleading with the laboratory director, you realize that you have no choice but to repeat the procedure.

You must now explain to John's parents that you are required to draw his blood yet again—and why.

Information and Preparation for the Standardized Patients We explain the situation to two confederates in the following terms:

> As John's parents you are extremely anxious and agitated, verging on uncontrollable anger. Your child has never been in the hospital and you are very concerned about his well-being. You believe the medical team is doing more harm than good by attempting all these blood draws. It is very frustrating having to hold him down while nurses and doctors stick him with a syringe. Each time, it takes up to half an hour to obtain his blood and another half an hour to calm him down. John is extremely tired and irritable and you believe nothing has been

done to make him better. He still has persistent vomiting and diarrhea. Why so many blood draws? When the resident comes in to tell you that he or she must repeat the procedure yet again, you are visibly frustrated and upset. You keep pushing to find out why, arguing that it must be a mistake—and who's accountable?

Learning Objectives We aim in this scenario to teach the importance of demonstrating accountability and evincing genuine empathy for the experience of parents and patients alike through an effort to respond honestly and openly when a mistake occurs and to explain that safeguard measures are in place to prevent a recurrence. For this scenario, we purposely chose an error that is not life-threatening but causes parents immediate distress and engenders anger, fear, and confusion. Apologies conveyed with appropriate openness and empathy, together with a professional but non-aloof demeanor, can effectively reduce anger and blame, help restore trust, limit antagonism, and have a positive impact on the future relationship (Garbutt et al., 2007; Robbennolt, 2009).

Case 2: Breaking Bad News Working in the emergency department, you are evaluating Jane, an 18-month-old toddler referred by her pediatrician's office for suspected new-onset diabetes. For the past week she has had polyuria, polydipsia, lethargy, and weight loss. Her dextrose stick in the pediatrician's office was 420. You have sent off the confirmatory lab work and indeed resolved the issue: she has type 1 (insulin-dependent) diabetes mellitus. You have called the endocrinology fellow and her team is on its way to assess the patient. You have given the patient appropriate IV fluids and insulin. Jane is currently stable with no complaints.

Jane's concerned mother has asked the nurse for an update several times. You must now disclose Jane's diagnosis.

Information and Preparation for the Standardized Patient

Ahead of this scenario we explain to a female standardized patient:

> You are a single mom. Your pediatrician has already told you there is a suspicion of diabetes. No one in your family has diabetes, and what little you know about the disease you've learned from television shows. You have seen people requiring limb amputations on TV as a consequence of diabetes. You know that Jane will probably need daily injections for the rest of her life but feel extremely afraid of the idea of administering them when she is so young that she can hardly talk. You do not think either you or Jane can handle that. You worry about Jane's ability to lead a normal life, go to college, and have a family. You are overwhelmed by the diagnosis. If asked, you wish to speak with a social worker to help you cope with the news. Your support system includes your own mother and your sister, and you ask that they be called.

Learning Objectives For this scenario we adopt the strategic protocol known as SPIKES, a practical and empathic method for communicating difficult or dire medical information to patients and family members (Baile et al., 2000). Developed in the late 1990s originally in the context of oncology, with the basic objectives of providing information and support and eliciting the patient's collaboration, SPIKES emerged from an earlier, broader investigation of how to deliver bad news in clinical context and has inherently wider applicability (Buckman & Kason, 1992). As we adopt it for a pediatrics setting, the strategy represents a useful stepwise mnemonic that can provide a basic framework for communicating with parents:

Setting: Arrange for privacy and quiet in circumstances where you and the parent or parents (and in some cases, the patient) can be seated, and seek to establish rapport.

Perception: Determine the level of comprehension and what the parent (or patient) knows or suspects about the medical condition, but at this stage do not confront denial.

Invitation: Ask if the parent wishes to know details of the medical condition, recognizing that some do not.

Knowledge: Use lay language that the parent can readily understand. Provide information using brief and uncomplicated sentences, offering any favorable assessments and positive details first. Avoid excessive bluntness and such phrasings as, "There is nothing we can do at this point."

Emotions: Identify the emotions presented by the parents and validate them, explicitly or implicitly. Respond by demonstrating, whether verbally or nonverbally, that you recognize and empathize with the way they feel.

Strategy and summary: Clarify any areas of concern and discuss treatment options; present an agenda for moving forward.

Case 3: The Angry Parent Mary and Jack are the parents of Nicholas, a 15-year-old male with trisomy 21 who has been admitted several times as an inpatient for multiple medical issues including a repaired atrioventricular canal, asthma, and constipation; he has also had behavioral issues.

Today Nicholas has been transferred to the pediatric intensive care unit (ICU) with left-sided pneumonia and empyema after 2 days in the hospital; he is being treated with intravenous (IV) antibiotics. Last night he developed moderate respiratory distress, with no improvement in cough and high fever. A chest x-ray showed worsening pneumonia and an ultrasound demonstrated an empyema. The surgeon has been contacted but has yet to assess the patient. Nicholas is currently receiving oxygen via a nasal canula and broad-spectrum IV antibiotics.

During morning prerounds, you hear Mary and Jack screaming at a nurse in a nearby room. They are visibly agitated, extremely angry, and almost threatening. Furious that Nicholas has yet to be assessed, they are demanding to speak to the chief of surgery. You enter the room to see what might be done.

Information and Preparation for the Standardized Patients We explain to the confederate mother and father:

> You are upset to see your son suffering and have become exceedingly angry and feel highly frustrated. Before Nicholas was transferred to the ICU, you were told a surgeon would stop by. That was 5 hours ago. You've grown progressively irate. You blame the team for Nicholas's decompensation and now believe they missed something. Moreover, you see no improvement in Nicholas's status since he's been transferred to intensive care and you are worried that nothing is being done for him. It is hard enough caring for a child with Down's syndrome and you are both taxed to the limit every day. Nicholas has required hospitalizations for other medical issues and taking care of him is a full-time job. You are both very tired. Jack works two jobs to make ends meet and Mary stays at home to take care of Nicholas and his three siblings.

Learning Objectives Parental fears concerning both iatrogenic harm and nosocomial errors during a child's hospitalization are well known and widely documented (Cox et al., 2013; Tarini, Lozano, & Christakis, 2009). We seek to help residents learn to understand parents' and patients' perspectives and, if necessary, to help them refocus expectations. Residents should be aware that the presence of the child may represent a danger in subjecting him or her to unnecessary stress (Coyne, 2006). In any acute illness, the pediatrician must frequently reassess the patient and update parents, validate their feelings, understand their anger, and remain aware of the importance of careful listening and nonverbal communication.

Case 4: Suspecting Child Abuse Erin, an 8-month-old baby girl, presents in the emergency department with seizures. Accompanying the mother, Janet, is her boyfriend, Carl. Janet is visibly upset and concerned while Carl nervously paces just outside the emergency bay while you are assessing and resuscitating the baby. Carl asks numerous questions about what is being done to the baby before growing angry and agitated, then storming out of the emergency department. You stabilize the baby and perform a computed tomography (CT) scan of her head. The radiologist calls you to notify you of multiple chronic and acute subdural hemorrhages.

Upon further questioning, you find out that Janet is a 20-year-old single mother working two jobs to support herself and her baby. She and Carl have been living together for 5 months. She was at work this morning and he was at home when she received his phone call. Erin, Carl told her, was "not acting like herself" and was extremely irritable. When she returned from work, she found Erin crying inconsolably, and after a time she showed signs of a generalized tonic–clonic seizure. EMS brought her to the emergency department.

You must tell Janet that you suspect child maltreatment and abuse and have an obligation to report your suspicions to the local or state authority.

Information and Preparation for the Standardized Patient We explain to the young female parent:

> You are extremely worried about Erin and traumatized by helplessly witnessing your baby undergo uncontrollable, spasmodic seizures. You are also upset that Carl angrily deserted you in the emergency department. You have never suspected Carl of abuse and leave Erin alone with him often because you work such long hours and he is on disability. You are shocked when the doctor voices what sounds like a firm accusation of abuse. You are confused and vulnerable, afraid for yourself and your boyfriend, and feel like you're in trouble and have been betrayed.

Learning Objectives Observations and data from radiology suggestive of abusive head trauma (Kemp et al., 2011) create conditions by which a physician has a medico–legal obligation and becomes a mandated reporter for suspected child abuse. Interaction with the parent should show concern for the patient's well-being and generate rapport that avoids accusations or judgment.

Extending Organizational Memory

For the communications program, our decision to use actual incidents as the basis for simulation scenarios represents a response to challenges in delivery of optimal care in a culturally diverse metropolitan health system. Addressing the various conflicts that affect patients and family members, concerning issues from parental authority and child-rearing practices to drug compliance, requires high levels of understanding, sensitivity to cultural norms, and skill on the part of interprofessional medical teams. As a means to educate residents and help them to develop those abilities, we thus draw upon our health system's organizational and "transactive" memory (Jweinat et al., 2013; Kransdorff, 2006). As we indicate below, we currently envisage extending this approach to help advance formative assessment.

Evaluation of Communication and Professionalism Domains

The ACGME's long-term program to improve graduate medical education dates to its 1998 Outcome Project and to further iterations, over the past 15 years, of its broader efforts to ensure competency-based education. Although the comprehensive character of the six domains of general competency (see Table 9.2) that the project outlines has been widely acknowledged, implementation into curricula for residents-in-training in the various specialties has developed as a complex, multifactorial, and long-term challenge. In spite of the Assessment Toolbox, a 2006 collaboration between the American Board of Medical Specialties (ABMS) and ACGME (Hicks et al., 2010), a decade later there was continuing "confusion and controversy about how to integrate the competencies into training in a meaningful way" (Carraccio & Burke, 2010, p. 419). The more recent "milestone projects" for the various specialties represent a further evolution of the original Outcome Project, and these are beginning to yield positive results as a way forward for residency education (Schumacher et al., 2013).

The Pediatrics Milestone Project, launched in 2009 as a joint endeavor by the ACGME and American Board of Pediatrics, provides a learner-based approach that specifies benchmarks and refines the six domains of competency as they apply to the specialty. Behaviors and attributes characterize each competency at specific levels of training and allow residents and educators alike to understand the knowledge, skills, and attitudes required to progress to the next level of proficiency (Carraccio & Burke, 2010).

Multisource Evaluation

What is the best way to evaluate the interpersonal and communications skills that pediatrics residents must acquire? It remains an open question. Recently, Brinkman and colleagues pointed out that assessment of such skills, with their inevitably subjective dimension, has traditionally been by supervising attending physicians, who may often evaluate residents concerning behaviors they have not actually witnessed, and there are in any event limitations of inferences when a physician assesses interpersonal behavior (Brinkman et al., 2006). They are among others to raise the prospect—and, indeed, provide an example—of using a multisource approach to develop evaluation procedures that make use of the Pediatrics Milestones in clinical context to further develop our communications program (Lockyer, 2003).

Multisource feedback (MSF), or 360° evaluation, was developed as a human resources tool in business and as a form of "peer evaluation" that has been used at times in medicine since the early 1990s (Ramsey et al., 1993). Its key advantage is to employ reliable formative assessment information from input supplied by multiple individuals operating from different perspectives. For purposes of pediatrics communication and professionalism, nurses, family members, and other residents would supply evaluations, not only the attending physician or faculty member. Research indicates that MDF "can contribute particularly to the development of behavior in more intangible domains of competence, such as communication, timeliness of completing tasks, taking responsibility, and professionalism" (ten Cate & Sargeant, 2011, p. 453).

We envisage a research-based effort to use 360° evaluation techniques to confirm whether and to what extent self-reported increased confidence—overwhelmingly positive in our postcourse evaluations—in the competency domains of communications and professionalism is warranted. We will develop a structure that requests input for individual residents from attending physicians, other residents, medical students, and nurses using an evaluative tool that aligns with the Pediatric Milestones. Evaluation during the first year of training, before residents take the simulation communication course, will provide a set of benchmarks that will be used to augment the needs assessment to highlight potential weaknesses of the trainee class as a whole. Once residents complete the course, they will be reevaluated according to the same methods as before. The overall objective will be to discover whether a focused communications and professionalism simulation curriculum based on an a priori needs assessment will result in reliable improvement of identified markers within the clinical environment.

REFERENCES

Baile, W. F., Buckman, R., Lenzi, R., Glober, G., Beale, E. A., & Kudelka, A. P. (2000). SPIKES—A six-step protocol for delivering bad news: Application to the patient with cancer. *The oncologist, 5*(4), 302–311.

Beaubien, J. M., & Baker, D. P. (2004). The use of simulation for training teamwork skills in health care: How low can you go? *Quality and Safety in Health Care, 13*(Suppl 1), i51–i56. doi:10.1136/qhc.13.suppl_1.i51

Brinkman, W. B., Geraghty, S. R., Lanphear, B. P., Khoury, J. C., Gonzalez del Rey, J. A., DeWitt, T. G., & Britto, M. T. (2006). Evaluation of resident communication skills and professionalism: A matter of perspective? *Pediatrics, 118*(4), 1371–1379. doi:10.1542/peds.2005-3214

Buckman, R., & Kason, Y. (1992). *How to break bad news: A guide for health care professionals.* Baltimore, MD: Johns Hopkins University Press.

Carraccio, C., & Burke, A. E. (2010). Beyond competencies and milestones: Adding meaning through context. *Journal of Graduate Medical Education, 2*(3), 419–422. doi:10.4300/jgme-d-10-00127.1

Cox, E. D., Carayon, P., Hansen, K. W., Rajamanickam, V. P., Brown, R. L., Rathouz, P. J., . . . Buel, L. A. (2013). Parent perceptions of children's hospital safety climate. *BMJ Quality and Safety, 22*(8), 664–671. doi:10.1136/bmjqs-2012-001727

Coyne, I. (2006). Children's experiences of hospitalization. *Journal of Child Health Care, 10*(4), 326–336. doi:10.1177/1367493506067884

Garbutt, J., Brownstein, D. R., Klein, E. J., Waterman, A., Krauss, M. J., Marcuse, E. K., . . . Gallagher, T. H. (2007). Reporting and disclosing medical errors: Pediatricians' attitudes and behaviors. *Archives of Pediatrics and Adolescent Medicine, 161*(2), 179–185. doi:10.1001/archpedi.161.2.179

Grant, V., Duff, J., Bhanji, F., & Cheng, A. (2013). Simulation in Pediatrics. In A. I. Levine, S. DeMaria Jr., A. D. Schwartz, A. J. Sim (Eds.), *The comprehensive textbook of healthcare simulation* (pp. 495–510). New York, NY: Springer.

Halamek, L. P., & Yaeger, K. A. (2008). Simulation in paediatrics. In R. H. Riley (Ed.), *Manual of simulation in healthcare* (pp. 337–349). New York, NY: Oxford University Press.

Hicks, P. J., Schumacher, D. J., Benson, B. J., Burke, A. E., Englander, R., Guralnick, S., . . . Carraccio, C. (2010). The pediatrics milestones: Conceptual framework, guiding principles, and approach to development. *The Journal of Graduate Medical Education, 2*(3), 410–418. doi:10.4300/jgme-d-10-00126.1

Issenberg, S. B., Chung, H. S., & Devine, L. A. (2011). Patient safety training simulations based on competency criteria of the Accreditation Council for Graduate Medical Education. *Mount Sinai Journal of Medicine, 78*(6), 842–853. doi:10.1002/msj.20301

Issenberg, S. B., McGaghie, W. C., Petrusa, E. R., Lee Gordon, D., & Scalese, R. J. (2005). Features and uses of high-fidelity medical simulations that lead to effective learning: A BEME systematic review. *Medical Teacher, 27*(1), 10–28. doi:10.1080/01421590500046924

Jweinat, J., Damore, P., Morris, V., D'Aquila, R., Bacon, S., & Balcezak, T. J. (2013). The safe patient flow initiative: A collaborative quality improvement journey at Yale-New Haven Hospital. *Joint Commission Journal on Quality and Patient Safety, 39*(10), 447–459.

Kemp, A. M., Jaspan, T., Griffiths, J., Stoodley, N., Mann, M. K., Tempest, V., & Maguire, S. A. (2011). Neuroimaging: What neuroradiological features distinguish abusive from nonabusive head trauma? a systematic review. *Archives of Disease in Childhood, 96*(12), 1103–1112. doi:10.1136/archdischild-2011-300630

Kransdorff, A. (2006). *Corporate DNA: Using organizational memory to improve poor decisionmaking.* Aldershot, England; Burlington, VT: Gower.

Ling, L., Derstine, P., & Cohen, N. (2013). Implementing milestones and clinical competency committees: Accreditation council for graduate medical education. http://webcache .googleusercontent.com/search?q=cache:t81Ay397Wb0J:https://www.acgme.org/acgmeweb/ Portals/0/PDFs/ACGMEMilestones-CCC-AssesmentWebinar.pdf+&cd=2&hl=en&ct=clnk& gl=us&client=firefox-a. Accessed July 1, 2014.

Lockyer, J. (2003). Multisource feedback in the assessment of physician competencies. *Journal of Continuing Education in the Health Professions, 23*(1), 4–12. doi:10.1002/chp.1340230103

Lorin, M. I., Palazzi, D. L., Turner, T. L., & Ward, M. A. (2008). What is a clinical pearl and what is its role in medical education? *Medical Teacher, 30*(9–10), 870–874. doi:10.1080/01421590802144286

Oshimura, J., Sperring, J., Bauer, B. D., & Rauch, D. A. (2012). Inpatient staffing within pediatric residency programs: Work hour restrictions and the evolving role of the pediatric hospitalist. *Journal of Hospital Medicine, 7*(4), 299–303. doi:10.1002/jhm.952

Peets, A., & Ayas, N. T. (2012). Restricting resident work hours: The good, the bad, and the ugly. *Critical Care Medicine, 40*(3), 960–966. doi:10.1097/CCM.0b013e3182413bc5

Ramsey, P. G., Wenrich, M. D., Carline, J. D., Inui, T. S., Larson, E. B., & LoGerfo, J. P. (1993). Use of peer ratings to evaluate physician performance. *JAMA: The Journal of the American Medical Association, 269*(13), 1655–1660.

Robbennolt, J. K. (2009). Apologies and medical error. *Clinical Orthopaedics and Related Research, 467*(2), 376–382. doi:10.1007/s11999-008-0580-1

Schumacher, D. J., Lewis, K. O., Burke, A. E., Smith, M. L., Schumacher, J. B., Pitman, M. A., . . . Carraccio, C. (2013). The pediatrics milestones: Initial evidence for their use as learning road maps for residents. *Academy Pediatrics, 13*(1), 40–47.

Swing, S. R. (2007). The ACGME outcome project: Retrospective and prospective. *Medical Teacher, 29*(7), 648–654. doi:10.1080/01421590701392903

Tarini, B. A., Lozano, P., & Christakis, D. A. (2009). Afraid in the hospital: Parental concern for errors during a child's hospitalization. *Journal of Hospital Medicine, 4*(9), 521–527. doi:10.1002/jhm.508

ten Cate, O., & Sargeant, J. (2011). Multisource feedback for residents: How high must the stakes be? *Journal of Graduate Medical Education, 3*(4), 453–455. doi:10.4300/jgme-d-11-00220.1

van Schaik, S. M., Plant, J., Diane, S., Tsang, L., & O'Sullivan, P. (2011). Interprofessional team training in pediatric resuscitation: A low-cost, in situ simulation program that enhances self-efficacy among participants. *Clinical Pediatrics (Phila), 50*(9), 807–815. doi:10.1177/0009922811405518

Yager, P. H., Lok, J., & Klig, J. E. (2011). Advances in simulation for pediatric critical care and emergency medicine. *Current Opinion in Pediatrics, 23*(3), 293–297. doi:10.1097/ MOP.0b013e3283464aaf

Four: Special Topics

Donna Marchant
Stanley Katz
Patti Adelman
Ronald Ulrich
Jane M. Wickey

10: Simulation Throughout: The Cardiology Fellows Program

The cardiology fellowship program of a tertiary care hospital employs simulation in an extensive and integrated fashion, both for purposes of instruction and for assessment. From their first day of participation, fellows experience high-fidelity simulation to ensure they are prepared to begin clinical work in the cardiology service. In sessions held throughout the 3-year program, fellows gain additional training using simulation with feedback for physical examination and diagnosis; they learn to perform transesophageal and transthoracic echo for both normal and abnormal hearts; and they practice the multiple skills required for diagnostic and interventional catheterization procedures. In addition, to help fellows improve their communications skills, and in alignment with current Accreditation Council for Graduate Medical Education (ACGME) recommendations, we have also designed a platform for Objective Structured Clinical Exercises (OSCE) with standardized patients who, together with faculty observers, provide post-hoc debriefings.

CARDIOLOGY AND SIMULATION FOR THE 21ST CENTURY

Training fellows in the multifaceted specialty of contemporary cardiovascular medicine is a long and complex endeavor. The broad aim, of course, is to equip specialists with the full range of imaging, diagnostic, and therapeutic capabilities and to provide hands-on instruction in the use of the ever-expanding set of interventions and procedures. Exceptionally rapid advances in cardiology, owing in great part to unparalleled success in detecting and treating heart disease, together with highly sophisticated tools and technologies, have created new and unprecedented challenges for faculty educators (Cates & Gallagher, 2012). The traditional apprenticeship model that relies largely on "hands-on" learning is today subject to increasing restrictions and more scrutiny, both in terms of patient safety and fellows' educational exposure to the whole range of patients, conditions, and clinical situations. In this context, simulation serves multiple purposes, takes place in several registers, and represents a paradigmatic change in teaching cardiovascular medicine in a postgraduate context (Marco & Holmes, 2008).

Although some recognized the future role for simulation in cardiology specialty training at the turn of the 21st century, it was not widely employed and its usefulness was by no means always or even frequently factored into educational curricula. The cardiology patient simulator (CPS) known as Harvey® had been developed at the University of Miami as early as 1968, and computer-based programs to run it were available by the late 1980s; it remains on the market today, distributed by Laerdal (Sajid et al., 1990). But its use in undergraduate medical education, clerkships programs, and various emergency contexts effectively preceded its usefulness for teaching cardiac fellows. In a "Perspective" piece for *Circulation* in 2002, for example, "Quo Vadis: How Should We Train Cardiologists at the Turn of the Century?," simulation goes unmentioned (Hill & Kerber, 2000). But just 2 years later, in 2002, the eminent cardiologist and then president of the American College of Cardiology, Douglas P. Zipes, discussed simulation as an "innovative education tool" and predicted that, "In the future, simulation training will revolutionize the way we teach, test, and treat" (Zipes, 2002).

Various factors might be adduced to explain the slowly evolving enthusiasm for simulation, including the exceptionally large skill set and knowledge base required for specialization, cost considerations, and advances in high-fidelity technology. Each of the various instances of outcomes-based research, although generally positive for a decade and more, tends to focus on specific tasks (Cates & Gallagher, 2012). At all events, in 2005 the ACGME devoted an entire issue of its bulletin to simulation, in which David C. Leach adduced ten reasons for its use in graduate medical education (Leach, 2005). By 2013 that organization produced a document specific to graduate training in cardiology, which mentions fellows' participation in simulation, although not as part of the "common program requirements" ("ACGME Program Requirements for Graduate Medical Education in Cardiovascular Disease [Internal Medicine]," 2013). A recent survey of ACGME programs indicates that, as of 2012, just about one in four interventional cardiology fellowship programs employed simulation (Green et al., 2013). Overall, gathering confidence in high-fidelity simulation generally, together with a small group of studies in areas that include catheterization and electrophysiology, has been more encouraging than decisive or game-changing (Bagai et al., 2012; Chugh et al., 2009). "The role of . . . advanced simulators in fellow training, postgraduate training, board certification and maintenance of certification in procedure-based fields," write Green and colleagues in 2013, "has yet to be clearly determined" (Green et al., 2013).

Increasing sophistication of computer-driven manikins, it should be noted, may play a significant role in adopting simulation for fellowship teaching in cardiology. Manikins' various built-in technologies enable them to mimic multiple pathologies, interact with diagnostic and monitoring tools, and react to interventions interactively with learners in real time. Since the turn of the century, no fewer than four endovascular simulators have reached the market and all provide haptic feedback (Green et al., 2013). Although experience clearly shows that the technology must be deployed in a structured way with feedback—as we discuss and emphasize in the following—the number of complex procedures available for learning through high-fidelity simulation is a recent advance (Cates & Gallagher, 2012).

Integrating Simulation With Fellowship Training

Our 3-year Cardiovascular Disease Fellowship at a tertiary hospital intensively and extensively trains fellows in all clinical and procedural areas. Components of the program include both clinical and basic science protocols in the context of in-patient service and ambulatory practice. Fellows treat patients from a wide range of ethnic groups and socioeconomic strata, and they acquire a full range of diagnostic, clinical, and procedural skills by which they progressively perfect their ability to provide care independently. Fully in line with the core competencies recommended by the ACGME, the 3-year program includes rotation through the various cardiac subspecialties (Table 10.1) and each fellow participates in some area of research. Our written curriculum, revised annually, provides for acquisition of a comprehensive knowledge base, and for all procedure-based rotations fellows achieve competency based on American College of Cardiology/American Heart Association joint guidelines.

TABLE 10.1 Cardiac Subspecialties Rotation

Coronary care unit
Clinical consultation service
Cardiac catheterization laboratory
Echocardiographic laboratory
Nuclear cardiology laboratory
Electrophysiology laboratory
Congestive heart failure
Cardiac computed tomography/magnetic resonance
Vascular medicine
Congenital heart disease

Introducing Simulation

We introduced simulation into our fellowship program in 2010, with a view to employing it as a complementary learning strategy. In collaboration with the Patient Safety Institute (PSI), we developed curricula for several high-fidelity simulation training platforms, each associated with specific educational aims: (1) the complete cardiovascular examination; (2) diagnosis by means of echocardiography; and (3) diagnosis and interventional procedures using catheterization. Each of these three platforms uses a different computerized manikin with distinct interactive features, and fellows train with them throughout the 3-year program. Beginning in 2011, in addition, we created simulation scenarios and a curriculum to help fellows improve their communications skills with both patients and colleagues; this program employs standardized patients. Fellows learn together in small groups and here, too, feedback and debriefing are constant features.

Physical Diagnosis

The cardiac physical exam—with careful history taking, palpitation, auscultation, and other maneuvers—is widely considered to be a declining art (Vukanovic-Criley et al., 2010). Reliance on the echocardiogram, which has become simple to perform and inexpensive, is probably in great part responsible for this de-emphasis; but it comes with a distinct downside when physicians fail to engage, for example, in the careful reasoning required for a sensitive evaluation of valvular pathology. Twenty years ago, Mangione and colleagues published results of a survey that showed an alarming decrease in auscultation taught in internal medicine and cardiology programs (Mangione, Nieman, Gracely, & Kaye, 1993). A decade later the same group showed significant improvement for internal medicine. But the issue remains one of concern today and an index of insufficient inattention to the cardiac exam, perhaps best understood as an artifact of the expanded knowledge base that the specialty requires.

Our use of high-fidelity simulation in conjunction with a postgraduate fellowship program calls for specific methodology and a caveat on assumptions about learning. It is our view that, through deliberate practice and in conjunction with clinical teaching, computer-based learning can help fellows perfect the various cognitive and tactile skills they require to meet current standards of practice. The manikin-based platform represents an extension of learning at the bedside that, although it makes use of sophisticated machines, at the same time serves as a reminder that the technology itself is not the unique vector for learning. Rather, simulation creates a unique set of heuristic relationships: (1) between learner and patient (manikin); (2) between learner and senior clinician; and (3) among learners, who learn from one another. Simulation is interleaved with clinical teaching at bedside and in office settings, with a view to full competency across the whole range of skills.

The physical exam with structured use of simulation offers a good illustration of these relationships. To help acquire proficiency in performing a complete cardiovascular examination—including inspection, palpation, and auscultation—fellows meet in small groups (usually four or five) at the PSI. High-fidelity simulation is preceded by didactic elements of the course, which include in-depth lectures on the physiology of heart sounds. For physical diagnosis the manikin is Harvey®. Fellows are each provided with a stethoscope microphone that enables them to individually hear and ultimately distinguish the various cardiovascular sounds in systole and diastole; they also learn to accurately detect heart murmurs. Initially the instructor (a senior clinical faculty member) performs the physical examination; subsequently, each fellow also auscultates the manikin while the others observe.

The simulator is able to produce in any order the distinct sounds of mild, moderate, and severe disease, enabling fellows to fine tune their listening skills over time in conjunction with their clinical work. They can learn the common sounds of chronic aortic regurgitation and chronic mitral regurgitation, but also the uncommon sounds of acute aortic and mitral regurgitation. With the manikin these sounds may be linked to the various other physical findings associated with these disease states. (With mitral regurgitation, for example: the cough, fatigue, shortness of breath, and palpitations can all be simulated.) Simulation sessions dedicated to physical diagnosis continue throughout the fellowship, with a view to the gradual assimilation and consolidation of the extensive knowledge base and skill set. First-year fellows attend five sessions; second-year fellows, four sessions; and third-year fellows, three sessions.

Simulation With Echocardiography

The wide variety of conditions that can be visualized and diagnosed in real time by ultrasound technology makes it an excellent training modality for use in the simulation laboratory with postgraduate fellows. In addition to aiding in diagnosis of heart failure, echocardiography can detect aneurysms and show enlargement of the heart (cardiomyopathy); it can also reveal anatomical conditions such as ventricular septal defect (VSD), and various congenital conditions such as transposition of the great vessels and tricuspid atresia. We use HeartWorks® (Inventive Medical Ltd.), a system that provides manikin-based high-fidelity ultrasound simulation. The interactive computer-generated model of the heart may be used to demonstrate both normal and pathological states, with anatomical relationships readily shown and demonstrated; display windows visualize both the three-dimensional anatomy of the heart and the corresponding two-dimensional image, both internally and externally.

Transthoracic echocardiography (TTE) is the most commonly performed ultrasound. High-quality images may be obtained at bedside and the procedure is essentially noninvasive, effectively pain- and risk-free, and comparatively easy to perform. It provides systolic and diastolic information, and can indicate pathology of the pericardium and valvular disease. Recently a randomized control trial supported the use of simulation to teach TTE to anesthesiologists (Neelankavil et al., 2012).

With simulation, junior fellows train in the basic scanning techniques and learn the various standard positions for applying the transducer to the chest (parasternal, apical, subcostal, suprasternal) and the multiple views they offer. They meet monthly with a senior fellow or attending physician with the aim of performing a complete transthoracic echocardiogram. Each fellow has the opportunity to be directly supervised as he or she performs the initial study. A recent upgrade that enables color and pulse-wave Doppler imaging allows fellows to perform and interpret more sophisticated operations.

Limitations of TTE—suboptimal images owing to obesity, for example, or pulmonary disease—may be overcome with the other principal mode of ultrasound for the heart, transesophageal echocardiography (TEE). As an invasive procedure that involves introducing the transducer into the esophagus, TEE is neither risk- nor necessarily pain-free. It is more challenging and demands further training in the use of the hand-held probe that provides, via computer monitor, high-quality contrast views (midesophageal, transgastric, and high esophageal) depending on level of intubation. Second-year fellows learn this procedure, also carried out with the upper-torso manikin, learning through simulation how to position and control the probe's flexion, rotation, and angulation capabilities. In addition to two small randomized control studies with anesthesiology residents validating the use of simulation to teach use of TEE (Bose et al., 2011; Jelacic, Bowdle, Togashi, & VonHomeyer, 2013), recent results of a similar study with cardiology fellows showed a similarly positive outcome (Damp, Anthony, Davidson, & Mendes, 2013).

Catheterization Procedures

Several studies indicate that simulators which reproduce catheterization in a safe setting augment the clinical experience of cardiac fellows (Bagai et al., 2012; Dayal et al., 2004; Green et al., 2013). Perhaps most importantly, the manikin enables focused performance and eliminates the stress associated with treating a real patient in a learning context, giving faculty the opportunity to instruct fellows without having to pay attention in real time to the patient's multiple signs and symptoms. As with other simulation modalities, it supplements and does not substitute for clinical work—although it should be noted that, as programming technology has advanced rapidly over the past several years, the faux patient responds to both proper and inadequate or failed interventions. Simulation may well prove to be cost saving if learners acquire the skills they need without compromising patient care; learning procedures on real patients may require less time to treat and fewer resources.

In 2010, the Center for Learning and Innovation (CLI) became the first facility in the nation to purchase Simantha®, a high-fidelity endovascular simulator that can be used as a supplementary platform to teach cardiac catheterization and endovascular procedures. Green and colleagues, who have reviewed this and several other manikin-based machines, noted its multimodal imaging and interventional capabilities together with its integration of ultrasound findings and hemodynamics monitoring. It can be used to assess cardiac, pulmonary, and cardiopulmonary disease. Scenarios involving acute diseases, which may be programmed with or without complications, create decision-making challenges for fellows: How would they manage the patient in terms of providing fluids, reducing blood pressure, or treating infection? Individual performance can be recorded and tracked over time.

As with other platforms, we use simulation for catheterization throughout the 3-year fellowship. In monthly meetings, first-year fellows learn how to perform a diagnostic cardiac catheterization and to understand and interpret hemodynamics during diagnostics. Second-year fellows continue this work but on patients with bypass grafts or other complications. Interventions are the focus for third-year fellows, including acute myocardial infarction and complications that can occur during various interventions.

Fellows also learn how to perform pericardiocentesis to aspirate fluid from the nondistensible cardiac sac, for which we have found simulation to be especially useful. Complications from this procedure owing to missteps in needle aspiration include pneumothorax, hemothorax, arrhythmias, infections, and arterial bleeding (Loukas et al., 2012). When done electively it is a high-risk procedure; when used to treat cardiac tamponade, it is a time-sensitive emergency that carries risk of death, all the more difficult to teach because it is infrequent (Tsang, Oh, & Seward, 1999). With simulation fellows learn the procedure and acquire the necessary tactile abilities together with use of hemodynamic monitoring, ultrasound imaging, and electrocardiogram. We scheduled pericardiocentesis simulation at the beginning of every month; interventional fellows orient junior fellows to the procedure and monitor their progress, with an interventional attending physician indirectly supervising the session.

Communications Skills

Cardiology fellows include a broad spectrum of personalities with disparate communications skills and styles. As physician specialists they will contend with an equally diverse group of patients and their families, and often in a context of life-and-death decision making. Not surprisingly, then, current ACGME Program Requirements demand that fellows be able to "communicate effectively with patients, families, and the public . . . . across a broad range of socioeconomic and cultural backgrounds" (ACGME Program Requirements for Graduate Medical Education in Cardiovascular Disease [Internal Medicine], 2013). They should also be able to interact effectively and efficiently with other physicians and health care professionals, and to function both as a team member and a leader. But how these nonclinical skills, not typically taught in medical school, should be acquired is not specified.

Operating in a large metropolitan health system with a high degree of diversity among both patients and personnel, we were powerfully aware of the problems associated with the complexities of patient interactions and teamwork when we inaugurated the cardiology fellows program. In 2011 one of us (DM) requested that the Center for Innovative Learning and its Physician Leadership Institute help address the interpersonal skills issues cited by the ACGME. The result was a further platform to our program at PSI that combines a self-assessment tool, group problem solving, simulation with standardized patients, and both individual and group debriefing.

Learning Through Self-Reflection In place of traditional didactics, we adopted an interactive and self-reflective approach. Prior to the initial session, fellows study a brief but concise summary of the Myers-Briggs Type Indicator® (MBTI), the widely used personality evaluation tool. The MBTI, rooted in the early theory of personality types originated by Carl G. Jung, was first published in 1962 and over the past half century, in the United States and the United Kingdom, has become widely used for team building, diversity training, and in a variety of other contexts, including health care (Allen, Brock, & ebrary Inc., 2002). It tracks normal, not pathological differences, and its modular structure makes it flexible and relatively simple to apply. It has proven reliability and a demonstrated level of validity appropriate to our heuristic aims (Kuipers, Higgs, Tolkacheva, & de Witte, 2009).

Working Through the MBTI In prereading and during our first session, we ask the fellows to assimilate the main ideas of the MBTI in an exercise that is both cognitive and involves self-assessment. We set out the indicator's global aim of discerning personality type in terms of preferences: how individuals distribute attention and energy; how they prefer to take in information and data; their style of decision making; and their orientation to the outside world. The heart of the MBTI is its set of four dichotomies (Table 10.2): extraversion/introversion; sensing/intuition; thinking/feeling; and judging/perceiving. Respondents choose one pole of each dichotomy. We ask the fellows to make their best-educated guess as to their own personality preferences.

Small Group Workshops With the aim of advancing from a theoretical examination of the Meyers-Briggs inventory to a functional application in terms of interactions with patients, families, and colleagues, we ask the fellows to work in small groups to discuss, synthesize, and teach back to one another the basic concepts of the MBTI. (The program director participates in these sessions.) We also provide the groups with a hypothetical case and ask them to apply what they learned.

Individual Sessions After completing the initial presentation and group discussions, we begin a series of observed simulations. Individual fellows enter into a consultation session with a patient and family members who are portrayed by standardized patients. We have developed two scenarios, both of which include powerful emotional components. One encounter involves a 76-year-old patient

TABLE 10.2 The Four Dichotomies of the MBTI

Extraversion	Direction of focus, source of energy	Introversion
Sensing	Ways of acquiring information	Intuition
Thinking	Ways of deciding and evaluation	Feeling
Judging	Preferred ways of interaction with the environment	Perceiving

CASE EXAMPLE: CARDIOLOGY ENCOUNTER

End-Stage Heart Failure–Home Hospice

Standardized Patient #1: Margaret Bailey, 70 years old (DOB 8/2/1944), is in bed, using a nasal cannula. She is relatively quiet throughout the encounter although she does react when conversation grows heated. She may be confused, even a bit frightened by the noise in the room. She does respond to the physician's questions.

Standardized Patient #2: Joseph Bailey, age 33, has been living at home looking after his mother, and is aware of the quality of her everyday life and her medical condition. Ron, his brother, has been sending money home to help care for their mother but the burden has fallen on Joe. Being so close to the situation, Joe understands that home hospice care is the best course of action. Having just gone through seeing his mother intubated/extubated he is convinced that "she should not have to go through that again." He is ready to bring her home with the help of hospice.

Standardized Patient #3: Ron Bailey, age 37, lives in Seattle and makes infrequent visits home but he is diligent about sending money each month and provides extra money when needed. This past week was his first visit in 2 months and to him "Mom seemed fine"; "She practically walked in here!" Although his brother has been keeping him up-to-date on their mother's condition, Ron does not understand how she could have deteriorated to this point so quickly. He wants the do-not-resuscitate (DNR) order rescinded and "everything possible done!"

Requisite Clinical Information for Fellows: *You will be meeting with the family of Mrs. Margaret Bailey (DOB 8/2/41), who is in end-stage heart failure. You are to discuss the need for home hospice with dobutamine.*

> *HPI: Recently admitted for respiratory distress and was intubated. Initial DNR rescinded by family. When patient was extubated, son Ron Bailey reinstated DNR.*
> *Critical aortic stenosis*
> *Previous bypass surgery 7 years ago*
> *Diabetes*
> *Hypertension*
> *High cholesterol*
> *Congestive heart failure*
> *Coronary artery disease*
> *Needs bilevel positive airway pressure (BiPAP) when sleeping*
> *Mild dementia*

whose clinical condition calls for a pacemaker but whose daughter is excessively demanding, condescending, and angry over what she perceives as inappropriate treatment. The other (see Case Example) is a case of end-stage heart failure in a 70-year-old woman, with family conflict and disagreement over the prospect of readiness for palliation and home hospice treatment. In each case, simulations last 6 to 10 minutes and are followed by one-to-one debriefs with the observer; these cover all aspects of the interaction, providing feedback that formatively assesses language, behavior, and presentation of self.

Group Debrief After all fellows have undergone individual simulation, we bring them together as group for a second debrief. Joining the fellows, attending physicians, and PSI facilitators are the standardized patients themselves, who explain the scripts they followed together with the cues and information, both in words and deeds, that they received from individual fellows, which shaped their own words and actions—whether provoking them to anger or ameliorating their initial hostile emotional stance.

CONCLUSION

Cardiology fellows are expected to master a wide range of abilities for both diagnostic and clinical purposes that require highly developed fine motor skills, specialized auditory training, and exceptional visual and tactile prowess. To ensure these skills together with the ability to communicate effectively with both patients and colleagues, we continue to incorporate both high-fidelity simulation and scenarios with standardized patients into our comprehensive cardiology fellowship program. We believe these efforts are consonant with a changing paradigm of postgraduate education in which simulation offers advantages in training physician specialists. Our use of simulation takes place in sessions throughout the 3-year program. We view simulation as both the right thing to do and plausibly cost effective if considered in relation to comparable efforts to teach at bedside. "Simulator training has the potential to deal very effectively with the apparently competing needs of training on the one hand and safety, efficacy, and timeliness on the other"(Kalman & Joseph, 2012, p. 1286). We agree and emphasize, as others do, that the full value of simulation arises not from the technology employed to teach fellows but in its use in conjunction with an experiential learning methodology with provision for continual feedback.

REFERENCES

ACC/AHA Joint Guidelines. Retrieved from http://my.americanheart.org/professional/Statements-Guidelines/ByTopic/TopicsA-C/ACCAHA-Joint-Guidelines_UCM_321694_Article.jsp

ACGME Program Requirements for Graduate Medical Education in Cardiovascular Disease (Internal Medicine). (2013): Accreditation Council for Graduate Medical Education. https://www.google.com/search?q=ACGME+Program+Requirements+for+Graduate+Medical+Education+in+Cardiovascular+Disease+%28Internal+Medicine%29.+%282013%29%3A&ie=utf-8&oe=utf-8&aq=t&rls=org.mozilla:en-US:official&client=firefox-a&channel=sb. Accessed July 1, 2014.

Allen, J., Brock, S. A., & ebrary Inc. (2002). *Health care communication using personality type patients are different!* (pp. viii, p. 213). Retrieved from http://www.columbia.edu/cgi-bin/cul/resolve?clio5636557

Bagai, A., O'Brien, S., Al Lawati, H., Goyal, P., Ball, W., Grantcharov, T., & Fam, N. (2012). Mentored simulation training improves procedural skills in cardiac catheterization: A randomized, controlled pilot study. *Circulation: Cardiovascular Interventions, 5*(5), 672–679. doi:10.1161/circinterventions.112.970772

Bose, R. R., Matyal, R., Warraich, H. J., Summers, J., Subramaniam, B., Mitchell, J., . . . Mahmood, F. (2011). Utility of a transesophageal echocardiographic simulator as a teaching tool. *Journal of Cardiothoracic and Vascular Anesthesia, 25*(2), 212–215. doi:10.1053/j.jvca.2010.08.014

Cates, C. U., & Gallagher, A. G. (2012). The future of simulation technologies for complex cardiovascular procedures. *European Heart Journal, 33*(17), 2127–2134. doi:10.1093/eurheartj/ehs155

Chugh, S. S., Donahue, J. K., Kaufman, E. S., Link, M. S., Markowitz, S. M., Narayan, S. M., . . . Group, C. F. P. D. (2009). The future of fellowship training in clinical cardiac electrophysiology: Program directors' perspective 2008. *Heart Rhythm, 6*(11), 1606–1612. doi:10.1016/j.hrthm.2009.07.044

Damp, J., Anthony, R., Davidson, M. A., & Mendes, L. (2013). Effects of transesophageal echocardiography simulator training on learning and performance in cardiovascular medicine fellows. *Journal of the American Society Echocardiography, 26*(12), 1450–1456. doi:10.1016/j.echo.2013.08.008

Dayal, R., Faries, P. L., Lin, S. C., Bernheim, J., Hollenbeck, S., DeRubertis, B., . . . Kent, K. C. (2004). Computer simulation as a component of catheter-based training. *Journal of Vascular Surgery, 40*(6), 1112–1117. doi:10.1016/j.jvs.2004.09.028

Green, S., Klein, A. J., Pancholy, S., Rao, S. V., Steinberg, D., Lipner, R., . . . Messenger, J. C. (2013). The current state of medical simulation in interventional cardiology: A clinical document from the society for cardiovascular angiography and intervention's (SCAI) simulation committee. *Catheter Cardiovascular Interventions, 83*(1), 37–46. doi:10.1002/ccd.25048

Hill, J. A., & Kerber, R. E. (2000). Quo vadis? How should we train cardiologists at the turn of the century? *Circulation, 102*(8), 932–936.

Jelacic, S., Bowdle, A., Togashi, K., & VonHomeyer, P. (2013). The use of TEE simulation in teaching basic echocardiography skills to senior anesthesiology residents. *Journal of Cardiothoracic and Vascular Anesthesia, 27*(4), 670–675. doi: 10.1053/j.jvca.2013.01.016

Kalman, J. M., & Joseph, S. A. (2012). Simulation and clinical training: The future and the indispensable past. *Heart Rhythm, 9*(8), 1286–1287. doi:10.1016/j.hrthm.2012.05.020

Kuipers, B. S., Higgs, M. J., Tolkacheva, N. V., & de Witte, M. C. (2009). The influence of myers-briggs type indicator profiles on team development processes: An empirical study in the manufacturing industry. *Small Group Research, 40*(4), 436–464. doi:10.1177/1046496409333938

Leach, D. (2005). Simulation: It's about respect. In A. Philibert (Ed.), *ACGME Bulletin* (pp. 2–3). Chicago, IL: Accreditation Council for Graduate Medical Education.

Loukas, M., Walters, A., Boon, J. M., Welch, T. P., Meiring, J. H., & Abrahams, P. H. (2012). Pericardiocentesis: A clinical anatomy review. *Clinical Anatomy, 25*(7), 872–881. doi:10.1002/ca.22032

Mangione, S., Nieman, L. Z., Gracely, E., & Kaye, D. (1993). The teaching and practice of cardiac auscultation during internal medicine and cardiology training. A nationwide survey. *Annals of internal medicine, 119*(1), 47–54.

Marco, J., & Holmes, D. R., Jr. (2008). Simulation: Present and future roles. *JACC: Cardiovascular Interventions, 1*(5), 590–592. doi:10.1016/j.jcin.2008.08.015

Neelankavil, J., Howard-Quijano, K., Hsieh, T. C., Ramsingh, D., Scovotti, J. C., Chua, J. H., . . . Mahajan, A. (2012). Transthoracic echocardiography simulation is an efficient method to train anesthesiologists in basic transthoracic echocardiography skills. *Anesthesia Analgesia, 115*(5), 1042–1051. doi:10.1213/ANE.0b013e318265408f

Sajid, A. W., Ewy, G. A., Felner, J. M., Gessner, I., Gordon, M. S., Mayer, J. W., . . . Waugh, R. A. (1990). Cardiology patient simulator and computer-assisted instruction technologies in bedside teaching. *Medical Education, 24*(6), 512–517.

Tsang, T. S., Oh, J. K., & Seward, J. B. (1999). Diagnosis and management of cardiac tamponade in the era of echocardiography. *Clinical Cardiology, 22*(7), 446–452.

Vukanovic-Criley, J. M., Hovanesyan, A., Criley, S. R., Ryan, T. J., Plotnick, G., Mankowitz, K., . . . Criley, J. M. (2010). Confidential testing of cardiac examination competency in cardiology and noncardiology faculty and trainees: A multicenter study. *Clinical Cardiology, 33*(12), 738–745. doi:10.1002/clc.20851

Zipes, D. P. (2002). President's page: Teaching: Today's investment in tomorrow. *Journal of the American College of Cardiology, 39*(2), 373–375.

Barbara DeVoe
M. Isabel Friedman
Kathleen Gallo

11: Strategy in Action: A Program for Nurse Retention

The Critical Care Nurse Fellowship Program, inaugurated in 2005, was designed to improve the retention rate for newly graduated nurses in the critical care units of two large tertiary care hospitals in a large and expanding health system. The structure and content of this initiative arose from two interrelated components: (1) an internal institutional reorganization that combined recruitment and education functions within the health system's corporate university and (2) an associated institute devoted to patient safety, operating under the aegis of that university. The rigorous year-long program employs a blended learning approach based on principles of adult learning that combine and align didactic online education with mentorship, preceptorship, and simulation. Subsequently, it has shown, as a result of improved retention and lower turnover, the sort of positive financial impact that may be expected to validate quality improvements to enhance patient safety.

We learned, in 2004, of high rates of turnover among critical care nurses at two large tertiary hospitals that formed the root of our large and expanding health system. Operating from a recently established corporate university that was charged both with implementing learning strategies throughout the organization and assuming the tasks associated with human resources, we were positioned to recognize the magnitude of the problem, to characterize it with respect to the nationwide nursing shortage announced about the turn of the century, and to create a comprehensive postgraduate educational program to improve nurse retention. Implementation of this program, as we detail it in the following, relied on a blended learning approach that activated basic concepts underlying the use of simulation for patient safety, including deliberate practice and debriefing, and preceptors who were trained to engage in critical thinking and develop an environment of mutual trust.[1]

HISTORIC CONTEXT

The postmillennial nursing shortage, as predicted, was different. With older nurses leaving the field and as many as six in ten new graduates leaving their first employment within 2 years, the numbers were startling and the situation unprecedented (Newhouse, Hoffman, Suflita, & Hairston, 2007). Job dissatisfaction was the key issue that best explained the early retirement of experienced nurses, declining numbers of nurse graduates, and overall difficulty in retention. Market solutions such as wage increases, which had worked fairly well in the past, "will not resolve the fundamental imbalances that plague nursing," wrote Eli Ginzberg, the economist who pioneered the field of career development, shortly before his death in 2002 (Berliner & Ginzberg, 2002, p. 2744). He pointed to the Nurse Reinvestment Act of that year as one step toward a solution and enjoined administrators and policymakers to "expand their vision beyond attracting more individuals into the profession."

The prospect of too few nurses in a sector as large and fundamental as health care led to a variety of assessments and proposed solutions to meet the challenges it created (Cavanaugh & Huse, 2004; General Accounting Office, 2001; Nevidjon & Erickson, 2001). Short-term efforts, such as hiring temporary staff or creating in-hospital agencies, were costly and raised concerns, especially in acute care settings, over patient safety (Lin & Liang, 2007). Not surprisingly, educational and training initiatives, cited by virtually all respondents to a 2006 survey, represented the principal long-term tactic on the part of hospitals and health systems. These included partnerships with nursing schools, subsidizing the salaries of nurse faculty, providing reimbursement in exchange for a commitment to work, and enabling nurses to attend classes (May, Bazzoli, & Gerland, 2006).

Special circumstances attended shortages in the fields of critical care nursing, where traditional recruitment patterns had undergone an important shift (Stechmiller, 2002). Almost six in ten U.S. hospitals cited critical care nursing positions as the most difficult to fill, with high numbers of vacant posts (Buerhaus, Staiger, & Auerbach, 2000). In the past, critical care nurses tended to self-select from the pool of experienced RNs, usually from within the hospital or health system. For the 21st-century nursing shortage, however, hospital consolidation and the passing of an older generation disrupted this pathway. In seeking to hire and train critical care nurses, health systems turned to the pool of new and recent nurse graduates. But here lack of experience, especially in the context of highly advanced critical care capabilities, including new technology and a growing intensive care unit (ICU) population, represented a clear area of special concern.

Responding to a 2004 survey of nurses at six Denver hospitals, for example, recent nurse graduates in acute care settings cited lack of self-confidence with respect to skills, including critical thinking; problematic relationship with both peers and preceptors; difficulty with dependency versus the desire to practice independently; and concern over their own organizational skills and ability to communicate with physicians (Casey, Fink, Krugman, & Propst, 2004). In brief, hiring nurse graduates to fill critical care positions was, in and of itself, likely to be an incomplete or deficient solution.

Formulation of a Strategic Initiative

The strategic purpose, concrete design, and administrative implementation of what came to be known as the Critical Care Nurse Fellowship Program (CCNFP) arose from structural changes to our health system that, in the final analysis, were based on principles of systems engineering and a thorough revision of educational content. In founding the Center for Learning and Innovation (CLI) as a corporate university in 2002, the administration assigned it the function of human resources, establishing linkages between educational initiatives and recruitment throughout the health system. As one result, we took first steps to develop the Patient Safety Institute (PSI), which would, by incorporating simulation and debriefing, generate greater and durable organizational awareness of the theory-rich content of adult learning.

When in 2004 we learned of severe shortages of critical care nurses in two tertiary hospitals in our health system, we were also aware that the difficulty in filling open positions mirrored the situation throughout metropolitan New York, where half of all new nurse graduates left their jobs before the end of their second year (Berliner, 2002). Our decision to create, in place of our standard orientation, a more comprehensive fellowship program for new hires in critical care units was consistent with cross-national findings, local conditions, and industry-wide recommendations (Aiken, Clarke, & Sloane, 2002; Maiocco, 2003).

Conceptual Foundations The basic components that defined the CCNFP all conformed to fundamental principles of adult interprofessional learning and collaboration. We included extensive online didactic course work, professional seminars, and provided fellows with nurse leaders as mentors and experienced critical care nurses as preceptors, with simulation as a learning strategy.

We should add that, as the foundational and overarching theoretical guide, we adhered to the stepwise model for nursing practice in the acute care setting, fashioned by Patricia Benner and based on the Dreyfus model of skills acquisition (Benner, 1984, 2004). In particular, we focused on three levels of skills acquisition that Benner investigated through longitudinal studies: (1) the move from reliance on abstract principles to the use of concrete experience; (2) the shift in perception of a situation in which all details are equal to a grasp of which parts are relevant; and (3) the advance from observer to participant.

However, the content of the program, and the interconnected alignment of its several elements—recruitment, online learning, use of simulation, and clinical experience—owed to adoption of a systems integration approach that aligned educational goals with the business of the health system itself (Dunn, 2013). It facilitated, in effect, development of a multiphased fellowship to improve nurse retention across a range of critical care settings.

Selection of Fellows Prior to developing the CCNFP, our standard program for recruiting and introducing nurse graduates into critical care units was comparatively extensive (May et al., 2006). Newly hired nurses received a standard 2-week orientation to the health system operations generally and to the specific hospital and nursing department to which they were to be assigned. They attended a 5-day critical care course with a core curriculum that consisted of lectures and assessment, with training in electrocardiogram (EKG) recognition, hemodynamic monitoring, ventilator management, critical care pharmacology, and stroke management. Each new nurse was assigned a clinical coach when starting work on his or her assigned unit. For the next 12 weeks they worked three 12-hour days per week and also took classes to introduce them to or improve their various critical care skills. Thereafter, at the conclusion of week 15, they were released from orientation.

For the CCNF, we built a high degree of selectivity into recruitment, in great part because the program was designed to be a more rigorous learning experience. We chose fellows—60 in 2007—based on qualifications together with the outcome of three separate behavioral interviews. After an initial interview with a talent acquisition specialist, the candidate would meet with the nurse manager who headed the specific critical care unit to which the nurse fellow would be assigned. We conducted a third interview at PSI, which included a description of the requirements and rigors of the program, including its academic demands and the use of simulation. Throughout we employed behavioral interviewing techniques that challenged candidates with a set of open-ended and situation-based questions that aimed to help elucidate relational and communications skills, judgment, commitment, and motivation (Bowen & Leger, 2013).

Program Components

The curriculum we designed for the year-long, tri-phase fellowship program was a blended learning experience that integrated didactic courses in critical care nursing with simulation and onsite clinical experience.

Titles and Nomenclature It was our intention that the nomenclature developed for the program would signal its nontraditional character and emphasize collegiality while avoiding potentially misleading connotations. Thus, we designated the nurse educator who followed each fellow's academic progress as a "master fellow," while the nurse who would traditionally serve as a fellow's preceptor, with whom he or she interacted on a daily basis, we named the "associate fellow." Beginning with the second phase, when fellows began work on their respective critical care units, we provided all parties with an "orientation contract" that detailed expectations and responsibilities. We emphasized the standardized character of the program to ensure that fellows understood their obligation was to acquire the competencies set out by each curriculum in order to be able to practice independently; it also outlined the collaborative team approach constituted by the fellow, associate fellow, and master fellow.

Preparatory Course for Preceptors We required the experienced nurses who served as associate fellows—they were selected by nurse managers—to attend a preparatory course that familiarized them with the role of preceptor as we at CLI defined and understood it. There we introduced them to principles of adult learning that many, if not most, would have known about only informally or through hearsay, if at all. We described simulation as a learning strategy, noting that as associate fellows they would serve as observers during scenarios and participate in the post-hoc debriefings. We outlined the concept of critical thinking as a skill for guidance and problem solving with respect to hands-on clinical activities, and we emphasized the importance of generating an environment of trust in which fellows would feel free to pose questions without fear of ridicule or reprisal.

Phase 1: Didactics and Simulation During the first phase (weeks 1 through 9), fellows work through the American Association of Critical Care Nurses Essentials of Critical Care Orientation (ECCO) program (Kaddoura, 2010). An online program, ECCO provides learners with modules that cover the whole range of critical care nursing: cardiovascular disease; pulmonary disorders; patients with neurological, gastrointestinal, renal, and endocrine diseases; hemodynamic monitoring; and multisystem disorders. The length of the phase, normally 9 weeks, is geared to the program's nine major topics; master fellows monitor individual progress. Weekly professional seminars complement and augment the coursework.

At the same time, in conjunction with ECCO, fellows attend simulation sessions that correspond to the areas covered in the coursework. The modular character of first-phase CCNFP is one of its distinguishing characteristics. While studying the cardiovascular component of ECCO, for example, fellows participate in simulation sessions concerning congestive heart failure and cardiac arrest and attend weekly seminars on such topics as cardiac rhythm recognition, EKG interpretation, and heart and lung sounds.

Phase 2: Shadowing and Clinical Pathway Fellows start their onsite clinical work (weeks 10 to approximately 26) by fully shadowing the work schedule of the associate fellow to whom they are assigned on a one-on-one basis. For each unit, a comprehensive critical care competency checklist and clinical pathway serve as tools, used by the nurse manager and associate fellow, in conjunction with the master fellow, to ensure the fellow's acquisition of skills. Although it might vary in content by unit, the basic checklist consists of detailed skills associated with all forms of devices and equipment, laboratory and diagnostic procedures, medication administration and pain management, and requisite competencies in the neurological, respiratory, cardiovascular, gastrointestinal, and genitourinary domains. Both the nurse fellow and associate fellow sign and date the checklist as it is completed.

Length of the second phase can vary somewhat depending on the individual fellow's progress and preexisting competencies.

Phase 3: Independent Assignments and Work Schedule From about Week 26 until graduation at 1 year, fellows function as independent practitioners and follow individual work schedules. A nurse educator onsite serves as an as-needed resource.

Measurement: Retention and Cost Savings

Sufficient data, deidentified and retrieved from information collected as part of the health system's ordinary activities, enabled us by 2007 to conduct a retrospective review that compared the retention rates for the CCNFP with the previous standard orientation of new critical care nurses, and also to provide a comparative estimate of associated costs. Our sampling frame consisted of two independent groups: all new graduate RNs hired during 2004 ($n = 30$), the year before the fellowship program was introduced, and the new CCNFP fellows for 2007 ($n = 60$). With this convenience sample, we were able to formulate two research questions: (1) What was the difference in rate of retention for new graduate critical care RNs, pre- and post-initiation of the CNFP orientation program? And (2), what was the net cost savings, if any, associated with retaining critical care nurses post-initiation of the CCNFP?[2]

To briefly reprise our findings, published in *Nursing Economics* in 2011, we found that annual retention improved from 53.4% in 2004 to 78.8% in 2007 (Friedman, Cooper, Click, & Fitzpatrick, 2011). We assessed the variables—age, length of employment, turnover—with measures of central tendency to ensure normality. In addition, we performed Chi-square tests on retention data at quarterly intervals: 3, 6, 9, and 12 months. The Chi values at all points except 6 months were statistically significant (Table 11.1). We suggest that at that point in the program, when fellows begin to share patient assignments on a one-to-one basis with associate fellows, they are especially apprehensive about their work and particularly vulnerable to issues around adequate guidance. During "bring back days" in the 3- to 6-month time frame, as we noted, fellows had an opportunity to provide feedback, and a recurrent theme was discontent with the associate fellow to whom they were assigned. Studies similar to ours have turned up similar observations, and these issues warrant greater consideration and more research (Morris et al., 2007).

TABLE 11.1 Chi-Square Values on Retention at 3 Months, 6 Months, 9 Months, and 12 Months by Program: Standard Orientation versus CCNFP

RETENTION (months)	χ^2	.
3	6.86**	
6	2. 4	
9	8.00**	
12	5.95*	

*$p < .05$, **$p < .01$.

To frame retention in terms of costs, we compared expenditures for recruitment advertising, which amounted to $488,596 (2004) and $166,995 (2007), for a cost savings of $322.501. Centralization of the advertising budget, previously generated separately by the two hospitals, could account for some savings. Although a comparison of turnover rates were not statistically significant between the 2004 and 2007 cohorts ($t = 1.22, p = 0.247$), the advantage in 2007 translated into the retention of ten more nurses, yielding a potential savings estimated at $1,367,100 annually—a financially significant advantage. With CCNFP, as with other learning initiatives, complexities arise in calculating the actual return on investment because benefits are "avoided costs" that are difficult to quantify, including quality of care, patient and physician satisfaction, impact of lower nurse–patient ratios, and burnout.

A Template for Nursing Fellowships

Generating the CCNFP through the offices of the corporate university and administering it on a continuing basis through PSI had the additional advantage of seeding other programs that deploy the same basic components: a core curriculum and blended learning experience, simulation, professional seminars, and an extended specially trained preceptorship for clinical experience. Using the critical care program as a template, we inaugurated the Emergency Department Nurse Fellowship Program in 2006 and, in 2007, the Pediatric Nurse Fellowship Program at Cohen Children's Medical Center. The latter program offered an opportunity to replicate our research with the CCNFP, with similar outcomes for retention, turnover, and cost savings (Friedman, Delaney, Schmidt, Quinn, & Macyk, 2013). We followed with inauguration of a nurse practitioner fellowship in 2012, a fellowship for nurses who work in the cardiac catheterization laboratory the same year (Palmer-Powell, Burns, Tanzi, & Floyd, 2013), and, in 2013, a maternal child nurse fellowship. To provide an iinterprofessional learning experience, emergency medicine residents participate in the simulation activities.

Multiphased fellowships such as the CCNFP represent one avenue to address the administrative and staffing problems created by the chronic and long-lasting nursing shortage. To cite the extensive body of evidence adduced by the Agency for Healthcare Research and Quality with respect to the impact of adequate nursing on patient outcomes (Kane, Shamliyan, Mueller, Duval, & Wilt, 2007), they also represent a strategic effort to improve patient safety and overall quality of care.

NOTE

1. The Critical Care Nurse Fellowship Program was renamed the William Randolph Hearst Critical Care Nurse Fellowship Program in 2007 due to a generous endowment from the Hearst Foundation. In 2011 the fellowship received additional financial support in the name of Rhoda Gilbert.
2. As indicated, we measured rates of both retention and turnover. Retention would be calculated as the number of RNs who remained in critical care divided by the total number at the outset, expressed as a percentage. The turnover rate refers to the percentage of RNs who left critical care divided by the number in the entire cohort.

REFERENCES

Aiken, L. H., Clarke, S. P., & Sloane, D. M. (2002). Hospital staffing, organization, and quality of care: Cross-national findings. *Nursing Outlook, 50*(5), 187–194.

Benner, P. (1984). *From novice to expert: Excellence and power in clinical nursing practice.* Menlo Park, CA: Addison-Wesley.

Benner, P. (2004). Using the Dreyfus Model of Skill Acquisition to Describe and Interpret Skill Acquisition and Clinical Judgment in Nursing Practice and Education. *Bulletin of Science, Technology & Society, 24*(3), 188–199. doi:10.1177/0270467604265061

Berliner, H. (2002). US healthcare. United straits. *The Health Service Journal, 112*(5811), 32.

Berliner, H. S., & Ginzberg, E. (2002). Why this hospital nursing shortage is different. *JAMA: The Journal of the American Medical Association, 288*(21), 2742–2744.

Bowen, M., & Leger, T. L. (2013). Interviewing job candidates: Behavioral techniques and tips. *Radiology Management, Suppl,* 33–37.

Buerhaus, P. I., Staiger, D. O., & Auerbach, D. I. (2000). Why are shortages of hospital RNs concentrated in specialty care units? *Nursing Economics, 18*(3), 111–116.

Casey, K., Fink, R., Krugman, M., & Propst, J. (2004). The graduate nurse experience. *The Journal of Nursing Administration, 34*(6), 303–311.

Cavanaugh, D. A., & Huse, A. L. (2004). Surviving the nursing shortage: Developing a nursing orientation program to prepare and retain intensive care unit nurses. *Journal of Continuing Education in Nursing, 35*(6), 251–256; quiz 278–259.

Dunn W, D. E., Maxworthy, J., Gallo, K., Dong, Y., Manos, J., Pendergrass, T., & Brazil, V. (2013). Systems integration. In A. I. Levine, S. DeMaria Jr., A. D. Schwartz & A. J. Sim (Eds.), *The comprehensive textbook of healthcare simulation* (pp. 95–110). New York, NY: Springer.

Friedman, M. I., Cooper, A. H., Click, E., & Fitzpatrick, J. J. (2011). Specialized new graduate RN critical care orientation: Retention and financial impact. *Nursing Economics, 29*(1), 7–14.

Friedman, M. I., Delaney, M. M., Schmidt, K., Quinn, C., & Macyk, I. (2013). Specialized new graduate RN pediatric orientation: A strategy for nursing retention and its financial impact. *Nursing Economics, 31*(4), 162–170; quiz 171.

General Accounting Office. (2001). *Nursing workforce: Emerging nurse shortages due to multiple factors.* Washington, DC: General Accounting Office.

Kaddoura, M. A. (2010). Effect of the essentials of critical care orientation (ECCO) program on the development of nurses' critical thinking skills. *Journal of Continuing Education in Nursing, 41*(9), 424–432. doi:10.3928/00220124-20100503-05

Kane, R. L., Shamliyan, T., Mueller, C., Duval, S., & Wilt, T. J. (2007). Nurse staffing and quality of patient care. *Evidence Report Technology Assessment (Full Rep),* (151), 1–115.

Lin, L., & Liang, B. A. (2007). Addressing the nursing work environment to promote patient safety. *Nursing Forum, 42*(1), 20–30. doi:10.1111/j.1744-6198.2007.00062.x

Maiocco, G. (2003). From classroom to CCU. *Nursing Management, 34*(3), 54–57.

May, J. H., Bazzoli, G. J., & Gerland, A. M. (2006). Hospitals' responses to nurse staffing shortages. *Health Affairs (Millwood), 25*(4), W316–323. doi:10.1377/hlthaff.25.w316

Morris, L. L., Pfeifer, P. B., Catalano, R., Fortney, R., Hilton, E. L., McLaughlin, J., . . . Goldstein, L. (2007). Designing a comprehensive model for critical care orientation. *Critical Care Nurse, 27*(6), 37–40, 42–34, 46–38 passim; quiz 61.

Nevidjon, B., & Erickson, J. I. (2001). The nursing shortage: Solutions for the short and long term. *Online Journal of Issues in Nursing, 6*(1), 4.

Newhouse, R. P., Hoffman, J. J., Suflita, J., & Hairston, D. P. (2007). Evaluating an innovative program to improve new nurse graduate socialization into the acute healthcare setting. *Nursing Administration Quarterly, 31*(1), 50–60.

Palmer-Powell, J., Burns, D., Tanzi, D., & Floyd, J. C. (2013). The evolution of a cardiac catheterization laboratory fellowship. *Journal of Continuing Education in Nursing, 44*(3), 103–104. doi:10.3928/00220124-20130222-03

Stechmiller, J. K. (2002). The nursing shortage in acute and critical care settings. *AACN Clinical Issues, 13*(4), 577–584.

Barbara DeVoe
Barbara Rhodes
Robert L. Kerner, Jr.

12: Dancing With the Stones: In-Situ Simulation for Lithotripsy

Hospital units that provide highly specialized procedures may benefit from in-situ simulation that enables observation under the identical physical conditions in which interprofessional teams work when responding to an emergency. Prompted by feedback solicited during debriefing after a laboratory-based simulation drill, an onsite high-fidelity program was developed to address potentially catastrophic events during extracorporeal shockwave lithotripsy in a dedicated unit. Deliberate practice during repeated simulations with a complete lithotripsy team demonstrated rapid improvement in teamwork in terms of communication and cooperation, including timing, physical movement, and both verbal and nonverbal interaction. Observation and debriefing of onsite simulation contributed to identification and on-the-spot remediation of latent risks and safety issues.

By custom and design, dedicated simulation centers such as the Patient Safety Institute (PSI) accommodate a wide variety of disciplines and operations. Convertible and modular, the settings for clinical encounters may be equipped as hospital rooms, operating rooms, emergency departments, intensive care units, and other facilities (Wheeler, Geis, Mack, Lemaster, & Patterson, 2013). Impression of fidelity is one of the defining features of simulation, even though the degree of requisite physical realism is an empirical aspect, ultimately subjective, which may vary with every scenario. Learning takes place through practice that involves, as Ray Page notes, "performing specific cognitive or psychomotor activities in response to stimuli indicating the need for such actions." Considering the experience in the aviation industry, he adds that fidelity "is limited by the weakest component producing stimuli" (Page, 2008, p. 45). When a dedicated simulation laboratory cannot provide sufficient fidelity to take the place of a complex hospital environment, in-situ simulation may be a solution.

Two basic advantages may be ascribed to improved fidelity for in-situ simulations, in which team training takes place on the actual patient care unit and for the most part uses that unit's equipment and resources (Wheeler et al., 2013). First, performance in the home environment may be expected to increase the psychological engagement of participants so that "fewer disconnects in the fidelity of the scenario occur because of unfamiliar surroundings" (Hamman et al., 2010, p. 227). In addition, and more importantly, in-situ simulation provides an opportunity to observe, identify, and correct latent safety or environmental threats (Patterson, Geis, Falcone, LeMaster, & Wears, 2013). Recent reports in the literature cite in-situ simulation with respect to tasks carried out in emergency units, labor and delivery wards, and a variety of other inpatient settings, including cardiac and pediatric intensive care units (see Chapters 4 and 8) and surgical suites (Garden et al., 2010; Miller, Riley, & Davis, 2009).

One might add that, in principle, if it were practical, simulation drills of all kinds might best take place onsite, where realism would not be an issue with respect to space and furnishings, resources and equipment, and whole team participation would be complete. But in general, although Forrest has set out basic guidelines for mobile simulation (Forrest, 2008), in-situ scenarios for patient safety, whether high fidelity or with standardized patients, are too prone to disrupt everyday activity in a hospital to expect they will become typical and widespread.

At North Shore University Hospital (NSUH), a large tertiary facility, the unit devoted to kidney and urinary stone removal employs the closed surgical procedure known as extracorporeal shockwave lithotripsy (ESWL). Providing a focused therapy that employs highly specialized technology, the lithotripsy team is interdisciplinary and its composition basically stable, with coordination and cooperation required for smooth operation. Still, unit personnel experienced the need to develop patient safety protocols in the face of potential adverse events. Viewed from a heuristic perspective, ESWL may serve as a stage for other similar hospital procedures that might benefit from onsite simulation. In the following we provide a stepwise account, structured to help provide a template for apprehending the potential for, and actually carrying out, in-situ simulations.

STAGE ONE: THE UNIT IN QUESTION

When it was introduced in the 1980s, ESWL revolutionized the treatment of kidney and ureteral (bladder) stones. For decades, stone removal from the upper urinary tract had been a full-scale surgical intervention. Device-based ESWL proved to be a disruptive technology that in most cases eliminated the need for a highly invasive procedure. With the lithotripter, electrically generated shockwaves propagate through water to pulverize calculi into fragments, which can then pass painlessly through the ureter. Originally developed by the airline industry for use in materials research, the lithotripter has proved to be a safe and effective alternative to open surgery (Doran & Foley, 2008). Today, although laser-based ureteroscopy can now treat small stones and percutaneous nephrolithotomy is still used for large calculi, ESWL remains the widely accepted standard. In the United States, it accounts for about half the procedures to eliminate renal stones (Pearle, 2012).

NSUH acquired a Dornier HM3 lithotripter in 1987 and developed a separate unit dedicated to treating urinary and bladder stones. Today the urology suite consists of a cystoscopy room for imaging, laser operations and stenting; a two-bed recovery room; and a separate procedure room that contains the apparatus for ESWL together with equipment for monitoring, x-ray, and patient transport. The Dornier HM3 occupies a fairly large footprint in a room that measures approximately 14 by 20 feet. The lithotripter consists of a large water bath, into which the patient is immersed, supported by a movable gantry with harness restraints, and the machine itself. In the following we provide further details concerning operations in the lithotripsy suite. Personnel present during procedures include the surgeon, full- and part-time perioperative RN nursing staff, a medical physicist (who operates the lithotripter), a perioperative assistant, and an anesthesiologist.

STAGE TWO: DETECTING SPECIAL NEEDS

Our first efforts to use simulation with personnel from the lithotripsy unit brought teams from the hospital to the PSI for typical high-fidelity code drills. These sessions were successful in terms of improving teamwork emergency response. However, during debriefing, and in response to pointed questions we posed as to whether these simulations were meeting the unit's needs, we received a candid response: They were not.

Both setting and team composition impeded fidelity of simulation. The physical setting at PSI could not adequately replicate the unique setup and complexities of the lithotripsy unit. How the patient was actually intubated and physically interacted with the lithotripter could not be addressed. In addition, the anesthesiologist, a key team member, was not present at code drills; nor was the surgeon. The verdict, developed as a result of debriefing, was clear. Inasmuch as simulation is about creating a realistic clinical environment, both globally and in detail, the drill was unsatisfactory.

We know that simulation initiatives may arise in a variety of contexts: through the suspected or projected need to implement protocol design, to improve team interaction, or in response to actual preventable errors and near-misses that led to delayed treatment with adverse outcomes, or for various other local reasons (Berkenstadt et al., 2008). In our case, we made the decision to employ in-situ simulation for the lithotripsy unit in response to constructive feedback from team participants.

STAGE THREE: SCOUTING AND RECONNAISSANCE

We visited the lithotripsy unit, watched and detailed the procedure, and planned for the transport of equipment, which would include a full-size manikin with monitoring capabilities and video-recording equipment.

Although in most cases ESWL is an outpatient procedure, it nevertheless usually requires full anesthesia. Some patients may also require preprocedure cystoscopy and ureteral stenting. In all cases that use the lithotripter, the patient is positioned on the gurney astride the water bath, sedated and intubated, then hydraulically lowered, unclothed, into the bath of degassed water.[1] Vital signs are monitored just as they would be during any surgical procedure. Physicians choose ESWL as the treatment of choice based on stone size and position as revealed by imaging. Except for small children and contraindications due to serious comorbidities, most patients can be cleared for this procedure, and for adults, age is not a factor, although there is a weight limit of 135 kg (297 lbs).

From the beginning we planned to simulate a cardiac or respiratory emergency while the patient was under sedation and immersed. Our manikin-based scenario was straightforward and planning for the simulation session followed a typical procedure. We developed a checklist (Figure 12.1).

STAGE FOUR: HIGH-FIDELITY SIMULATION

Preliminaries attendant to lithotripsy actually set the stage for simulation with a view to improving reaction time in the event of an emergency; they also outline and indeed underscore the difficulties inherent in emergency response during ESWL. From beginning to end, the procedure involves the entire team and follows some distinctive choreography. Various activities and elements, such as the stretcher transfer of the patient, would be uncomplicated and stereotypical if it were not for the architecture of the lithotripter. Although occasionally a patient is ambulatory and can help place himself or herself on the gantry prior to anesthesia and immersion, most start from the stretcher. With the medical physicist to one side of the patient and the surgeon on the other, the anesthesiologist holds the patient's head and the perioperative nurse, the feet. After coordinated transfer from the stretcher, the patient must be positioned so that the kidney area will be exposed; the patient's head is adjusted, then strapped into the gurney. The perioperative nurse first secures straps across the calves, then moves to help position the head. The medical physicist secures the safety straps across the chest, abdomen, and legs. He then positions the metal head rest and the head itself is secured to it by tape. Headphones are fitted over the ears to protect the patient from the sound the shockwaves make. A final top piece secures the intravenous (IV) tubing, the electrocardiogram (EKG), the blood pressure cord, and the pulse oximeter cord together with the wires for the anesthesia circuit and breathing tube that connects to the respirator.

These safety preliminaries conclude when the patient, positioned with all apparatus secured on the gantry, is hydraulically escorted to the water tub by the medical physicist, who turns the body from a north–south to an

TABLE 12.1 In-Situ Planning Checklist

Agenda

- In-situ overview
  - full staff commitment needed: MD, RN, perioperative nurse educator
  - clinical uniform, name tags, and so on.

- Scheduling
  - When do we want to target start?
  - Day of week?
  - How many sessions?
  - Target end date?
  - Length of session: How many hours?
  - Cancelation procedure?

- Subject matter of each simulation: What types of cases?
  - Who will be point person for developing the case?
  - Who is point person for the day-of activities?
  - Who will be the perioperative nurse educator?

- Number of participants per session

- Logistics
  - where: lithotripsy unit
  - debrief space
  - Will there be "watchers"? Where will they stage and what will they do while the case is running?
    - If yes, they need a room with a TV (VGA connection and audio).

- Use of meds, consumables
  - use their code cart, alert that they will need to restock
  - check their defibrillator for interface cables to Sim man
  - IV fluids
  - check for appropriate airway, intubation equipment, and clinical supplies

- Will there be anything else going on, on the unit?
  - distractions
  - inadvertent capture on video

- Involvement of other hospital staff
  - respiratory
  - anesthesia

- How many PSI staff will be needed?

- Metrics
  - Is there something we can measure/assess outcomes?
  - need CLI programmatic evaluation

- Manikin and simulation equipment
  - video capabilities
  - wireless
  - How long will it take to set up?
  - Does manikin need to cry, bleed (fluids)?
  - Portable monitor

- Parking logistics
  - Where to park ambulance?

east–west position, then lowers the patient into the bath until the water reaches the level of the breast. Using fluoroscopy, the physicist identifies the position of the target stone, which now becomes a focal point for the shockwaves—and the procedure begins. The shockwaves emitted from the bottom of the tub surge through the water, encounter the stone and degrade it, then dissipate at the surface. From 2,000 to 3,000 shock waves may be required to successfully fragment a typical stone (Doran & Foley, 2008).

We initially ran the simulation activity over the course of a full day. Sudden arrhythmia prompted the anesthesiologist to initiate the code and we timed the reaction of the team: How long did it take to recognize the potential emergency, halt the procedure, safely lift the patient out of the water bath, remove the patient from the gantry, make the transfer to the stretcher, dry the patient off, apply the pads and begin to defibrillate? Simultaneously, the team needed to call for the hospital's code team and procure the crash cart. Debriefings enabled the team to verbalize the various difficulties they encountered and set a course of immediate remediation through deliberate practice.

STAGE FIVE: PRINCIPAL FINDINGS AND DISCUSSION

We observed multiple missteps during the initial simulation drills. In attempting to remove the patient from the lithotripter water bath, people initially talked over one another, physically bumped up against one other, and in other ways interfered with each another's movements. Problems arose owing to the constraints of space around the machine. The clear outcome was significantly suboptimal response time. In terms of effective action in the face of an unforeseen emergency, in-situ simulation in lithotripsy revealed essentially a variety of small errors and missteps. Together they amounted to a latent environmental threat that we might describe with greater specificity as a *failure of reverse choreography*.

Coincident with and counterbalancing these issues observed during the early iterations of the simulation drill were several relevant positive factors. Although the anesthesiologist changes daily through service rotation, the lithotripsy team is basically stable. For the actual procedure, members work with a shared mental model and engage in closed-loop communication that helps them to follow protocol and, under normal circumstances, ensure patient safety. Obliged to coordinate their efforts, they efficiently orchestrate the progression to shockwave therapy and they build in backup behaviors and various task strategies into their movements. Operating in a closed space without distractions or interference from outside personnel, they tend to cooperate and develop a good measure of camaraderie and social cohesion. These elements of teamwork constituted a good basis for the immediate remediation.

Translating team competencies to the emergency response realm thus became the primary goal of the simulation exercise. From the beginning, all members were prepared to take on their respective roles during simulation and, indeed, they acted under the direction of the anesthesiologist, chose a leader to direct the code procedures, and carried them out—albeit with missteps at first. But in repeated simulation exercises in concert with immediate post-hoc debriefs, the registered nurses, perioperative personnel, anesthesiologist, and surgeon refined their behaviors. From an observational standpoint, the rescue procedure became smoother. Response time, the only reasonable metric in this case, significantly improved. We subsequently scheduled further simulations and planned to include drills for stroke and respiratory emergency.

If we apply guidelines such as those currently suggested in the literature, we can develop revealing pictures of the kinds of latent errors that in-situ simulation is able to detect and, also, in some cases at least, develop efficient on-the-spot remediation. Salas et al., for example, suggest patient safety relies on shared cognition and promotes a "three-pronged" approach to teamwork involving communication, coordination, and cooperation (Salas, Wilson, Murphy, King, & Salisbury, 2008). This approach has a good fit with others suggested over the past two decades, both within medicine and with respect to team training generally (Eppich, Howard, Vozenilek, & Curran, 2011; Guzzo & Salas, 1995; Mickan & Rodger, 2005). Subject to further refinement, these fundamental ideas underlying simulation serve the larger aim of developing a sustainable culture of patient safety. We can view that culture in microcosm in the lithotripsy unit.

NOTE

1. All patients are offered a disposable bathing suit; a one-piece for males and a two-piece for females. Direct access to the flank area being treated is an important aspect of the ESWL procedure.

REFERENCES

Berkenstadt, H., Haviv, Y., Tuval, A., Shemesh, Y., Megrill, A., Perry, A., . . . Ziv, A. (2008). Improving handoff communications in critical care: Utilizing simulation-based training toward process improvement in managing patient risk. *Chest, 134*(1), 158–162. doi:10.1378/chest.08-0914

Doran, O., & Foley, B. (2008). Acute complications following extracorporeal shock-wave lithotripsy for renal and ureteric calculi. *Emergency Medicine Australasia, 20*(2), 105–111. doi:10.1111/j.1742-6723.2008.01065.x

Eppich, W., Howard, V., Vozenilek, J., & Curran, I. (2011). Simulation-based team training in healthcare. *Simul Healthc, 6*(Suppl.), S14–S19. doi:10.1097/SIH.0b013e318229f550

Forrest, F. C. (2008). Mobile simulation. In R. H. Riley (Ed.), *Manual of simulation in healthcare* (pp. 25–33). New York, NY: Oxford University Press.

Garden, A. L., Mills, S. A., Wilson, R., Watts, P., Griffin, J. M., Gannon, S., & Kapoor, I. (2010). In situ simulation training for paediatric cardiorespiratory arrest: Initial observations and identification of latent errors. *Anaesthesia and Intensive Care, 38*(6), 1038–1042.

Guzzo, R. A., Salas, E. (1995). *Team effectiveness and decision making in organizations.* San Francisco, CA: Jossey-Bass.

Hamman, W. R., Beaudin-Seiler, B. M., Beaubien, J. M., Gullickson, A. M., Orizondo-Korotko, K., Gross, A. C., . . . Lammers, R. (2010). Using in situ simulation to identify and resolve latent environmental threats to patient safety: Case study involving operational changes in a labor and delivery ward. *Quality Management in Health Care, 19*(3), 226–230. doi:10.1097/QMH.0b013e3181eb1452

Mickan, S. M., & Rodger, S. A. (2005). Effective health care teams: A model of six characteristics developed from shared perceptions. *Journal of Interprofessional Care, 19*(4), 358–370. doi:10.1080/13561820500165142

Miller, K., Riley, W., & Davis, S. (2009). Identifying key nursing and team behaviours to achieve high reliability. *Journal of Nursing Management, 17*(2), 247–255. doi:10.1111/j.1365-2834.2009.00978.x

Page, R. (2008). Lessons from aviation simulation. In R. H. Rile (Ed.), *Manual of simulation in healthcare* (pp. 37–50). New York, NY: Oxford University Press.

Patterson, M. D., Geis, G. L., Falcone, R. A., LeMaster, T., & Wears, R. L. (2013). In situ simulation: Detection of safety threats and teamwork training in a high risk emergency department. *BMJ Quality and Safety, 22*(6), 468–477. doi:10.1136/bmjqs-2012-000942

Pearle, M. S. (2012). Shock-wave lithotripsy for renal calculi. *The New England Journal of Medicine, 367*(1), 50–57. doi:10.1056/NEJMct1103074

Salas, E., Wilson, K. A., Murphy, C. E., King, H., & Salisbury, M. (2008). Communicating, coordinating, and cooperating when lives depend on it: Tips for teamwork. *Joint Commission Journal on Quality and Patient Safety, 34*(6), 333–341.

Wheeler, D. S., Geis, G., Mack, E. H., Lemaster, T., & Patterson, M. D. (2013). High-reliability emergency response teams in the hospital: Improving quality and safety using in situ simulation training. *BMJ Quality and Safety, 22*(6), 507–514. doi:10.1136/bmjqs-2012-000931

Kristy Loewenstein
Marybeth McManus

13: *"Don't Tell Me to Calm Down!"* De-Escalation of the Agitated Patient in a Hospital Setting

Agitated patients require immediate intervention to avoid harm to themselves or others. Traditional methods of de-escalation in behavioral health, which invoke the use of physical restraint and/or involuntary medication, are freighted with undesirable consequences. A noncoercive approach, based on the emergent concepts of trauma-informed care, offers multiple advantages for patients and caregivers alike. This chapter details a clinical skills simulation program that employs standardized patients, immediate debriefing, and auxiliary teaching aids to help mental health professionals acquire and improve the skills they need to communicate with, constructively engage, and console patients in states of extreme agitation and aggression.

The management of aggression is a problem of interest in mental health nursing. Aggression may be physical (directed at self, others, or property) or verbal and, if not de-escalated, can result in restraint or seclusion of the patient and even in staff or patient injuries. Nursing staff and other mental health professionals are expected to be skilled in identifying imminent dangerousness and predicting the potential for future violence; they play an important role in identifying risk factors and implementing interventions that promote and maintain safety (American Psychiatric Nurses Association [APNA], 2008). Psychiatric health care providers experience high rates of workplace violence, yet little is known about the strategies that various facilities employ to reduce it (Peek-Asa et al., 2009). In response to the pressure of regulatory agencies, most psychiatric facilities now require formal education for nursing staff, usually on a yearly basis, to help manage aggressive behavior; but little is publicly known about the results these programs achieve (Morrison & Carney-Love, 2003). The APNA Position Statement (2008, p.35) notes: "To date, there are no national standards for staff training in the prevention and management of inpatient violence. Given the scope and significance of inpatient violence, it is both curious and troubling that staff training programs vary widely in content and process and tend to lack a consistently scholarly and empirical base."

AGGRESSION AND RELATED DEFINITION

Aggression is defined as any behavior, physical or verbal, intended to cause harm to another person or to oneself (enotes.com, 2010.) *Restraint* is any manual method, physical or mechanical device, material, or equipment that immobilizes or reduces the ability of a patient to move his or her arms, legs, body, or head freely (New York State Office of Mental Health [NYS OMH], 2007). *Seclusion* is defined as the involuntary confinement of a person alone in a room or area from which the patient is physically prevented from leaving (NYS OMH, 2007). *Physical intervention* is a skilled manual, or hands-on, method of physical restraint implemented by trained individuals, with the intention of controlling the aggressive patient, to restore safety in the clinical environment (Stubbs et al., 2009). *Staff attitudes* are the behavior and perceptions of staff members about the aggressive patient and the use of physical intervention or restraint/seclusion. *Patient perceptions* are feelings reported by patients about the act of restraint/seclusion.

We describe in the following the development of a verbal de-escalation program that employs simulation with standardized patients (SPs) in the context of a specially designed curriculum to help unlicensed assistive personnel (UAP) contend with agitated patients at risk for violent behavior. Our goal, to establish and maintain a restraint- and seclusion-free environment, is rooted in ongoing efforts to provide optimal care, employ patient-focused interventions, and adhere to the emergent model of trauma-informed care and recovery.

The Setting

Zucker Hillside Hospital (ZHH) is a 221-bed behavioral health facility that serves people throughout the five boroughs of New York City and Long Island who suffer from mental illness and/or substance abuse. The hospital's Behavioral Health Pavilion, which opened in 2013 and houses six of its ten inpatient units and the electroconvulsive therapy (ECT) suite, was conceived as a therapeutic environment with space and design elements to facilitate healing and recovery. The hospital offers a full range of services for patients, including adolescents and seniors. Its interdisciplinary teams include nurses, nurse practitioners, psychiatrists, psychologists, social workers, mental health workers, psychiatric assistants, rehabilitation and activity therapists, nutritionists, and pharmacists. The nursing department at ZHH has a strong commitment to quality measures and every staff member is trained in the TeamSTEPPS® approach and aggression prevention techniques for verbal de-escalation and personal safety. Safety of patients and staff is paramount and prevention and management of crisis situations, including agitation and aggression, are of utmost importance in maintaining a safe environment. But these tasks are difficult to accomplish and represent a constant challenge as we strive to establish a restraint- and seclusion-free environment.

Managing Aggressive Behavior: General Considerations

Incidents of patient aggression and violence are associated with inadequate staff training and organizational problems (Duxbury, 2002). Most psychiatric facilities implement some kind of formal education concerning the management of aggression (Duxbury, 2002; Farrell & Cubit, 2005; Godin, Smith, Cyr, & Finch, 2003; Irwin, 2006; Lepping et al., 2009; Martin & Daffern, 2006; Morrison & Carney-Love, 2003; Peek-Asa et al., 2009). In light of regulatory guidelines, many institutions now mandate annual training for nursing staff; however, the requirement to train personnel has resulted in a "small cottage industry of mental health consultants selling a program based on martial arts, and not all are based on sound professional and clinical principles" (Morrison & Carney-Love, 2003, p. 147). As a consequence, choosing which aggression management program to teach is by no means straightforward. As noted, little is publicly known with respect to outcomes and efficacy and there are no national standards for staff training (APNA, 2008). Hospitals and researchers have made efforts, however, to evaluate and sometimes to compare programs. Riverview Hospital, in British Columbia, Canada, for example, has adopted the Non-Violent Crisis Intervention® (NVCI) training from the Crisis Prevention Institute (CPI). They reported that the majority of staff felt more confident in returning to the workplace to deal with difficult behaviors after training (Godin, Smith, Cyr, & Finch, 2003). Peek-Asa and colleagues (2009) reviewed workplace violence prevention programs (WVPs) in California and New Jersey, compared the programs to each other, and evaluated how well they met state (California Occupational Safety and Health Administration [CalOSHA]) and federal (Federal OSHA) regulations. Noting that components of both included training, policy and procedures, environmental control, and security, they found that no WVP training programs in either state included all the components specified by law and concluded that "a comprehensive approach . . . is likely to be achieved only through multidisciplinary and representative input from the staff and management" (Peek-Asa et al., 2009). Similarly, Morrison and Carney-Love (2003) appraised four commercially available programs for the management of aggression in psychiatric settings: The Mandt System®, NVCI, Professional Assault Response Training (PART™) and Therapeutic Options™ (TO). They evaluated the content, feasibility (ease of use), psychological comfort of the staff (confidence after training), program effectiveness, and cost. TO and PART, they found, met most of their criteria; they rated CPI and Mandt somewhat lower. Using different criteria, Farrell and Cubit (2005) assessed 28 programs available in Australia, including the four evaluated by Morrison and Carney-Love (2003). They listed components but did not score or rate them. Categories included orientation to the workplace, causes and types of aggression, and legal and ethical concepts, to name several. A program called CIPO—Critical Incident Positive Outcome, from the Rozelle Hospital in Australia—met the most criteria (11 of 12). Of four programs also considered by Morrison and Carney-Love (2003), CPI met 7 out of 12 criteria; PART, 6 of 12; Mandt, 7 of 12; and TO, 5 of 12. Both studies suggest that training programs should include regulatory guidelines together with the psychological and organizational costs associated with aggression; in addition, they ought to be comprehensive, with managerial support being integral to success (Morrison & Carney-Love, 2003; Farrell & Cubit, 2005). At ZHH, we developed our own crisis prevention course, today known as Aggression Prevention Training (APT). Developed by Peter D'Amico, PhD (D'Amico, Kim, & Stephens 2008), the hospital's director of child and adolescent psychology, APT is only available in the North Shore–LIJ (NS-LIJ) health system. Based on the curriculum promulgated by New York State's Office of Mental Health (OMH) for Preventing and Managing Crisis Situations (PMCS), it includes elements of dialectical behavior therapy and other therapeutic behavioral techniques, including validating the patient's feelings.[1]

Regardless of the program used to train staff, major shared components include theory and the conceptual structures for understanding violence and aggression; prevention, or assessment of danger and taking precautions; and interaction with the patient and post-incident action, which includes reporting, investigating, and counseling (Farrell & Cubit, 2005). At the very least, training can increase staff members' confidence in their ability to handle aggressive or violent situations (Martin & Daffern, 2006). A European study of perceived ward safety found that in Britain 91% of ward managers confirmed that their staff had completed training regarding violent incidents, compared to 68% in Germany and 60% in Sweden (Lepping et al., 2009). The British managers, whose hospitals also had the highest staffing levels per patient, viewed violence and aggression as less problematic.

Patient-Focused Interventions

Behavior plans, when implemented consistently and with multidisciplinary collaboration and cooperation, can result in decreased incidence of aggression and a reduction in the need to use restrictive interventions to manage aggression. A 2006 case study (Bisconer, Green, Mallon-Czajka, & Johnson, 2006) found that the implementation of a plan that took into consideration the subject's problems, goals, target behaviors (both to augment and reduce), and reinforcers, together with staff training, were able to help the patient require fewer restrictive interventions and reduce the number of incidents of physical aggression toward self and others. Other research has outlined how an Individual Crisis Prevention Plan can be a useful tool to assist patients in regaining control by utilizing specific strategies, identified by the patient as soothing or calming (Champagne & Stromberg, 2004; NYS OMH 2007). Individual crisis plans should be written with the patient, not for the patient. The patient needs to identify his or her "triggers" to aggression or self-injury, and what helps him or her regain control. Some patients, for example, may listen to headphones to mitigate the sound of the voices they are hallucinating; others may be able to watch television or read a book. Sensory approaches, such as aromatherapy, therapeutic touch, squeezing a stress ball, or watching a fish in an aquarium sometimes help a person to regain control as well as avoid the need for restraint or seclusion (Champagne & Stomberg, 2004).

Various other patient-focused interventions to contend with aggressive behavior have also been described. Core themes identified by nurses in the Hertfordshire/Oxfordshire Violent Incident Study (Spokes et al., 2002) included interpersonal skills combined with clinical skills and personal characteristics. These skills, "in particular in relation to abilities in communication and in the development of relationships . . . may be considered the most important staff factors as they relate to the development of therapeutic relationships that are central to the clinical role in nursing" (p. 205). Along quite similar lines, as we discuss in more detail in the following, trauma-informed care—that is, care that addresses the significant effect that trauma may have on a person—can be crucial to understanding and preventing aggression in behavioral health hospital settings (Champagne & Stromberg, 2004).

Trauma-Informed Care and the Recovery Model

In general, current efforts in psychiatric facilities to reduce or eliminate seclusion and restraint owe in part to the emerging values of the trauma-informed care movement. A "trauma-informed" facility designs systems that accommodate vulnerabilities of trauma survivors and delivers services in ways that will facilitate consumer participation in treatment and avoid inadvertent retraumatization (Jennings, 2007). The PMCS curriculum, as discussed, aims to develop trauma-centered care that creates an Individual Crisis Prevention Plan for each patient, and reviews restraint and seclusion, regulatory and legal ramifications, and debriefing of staff and patients, with physical intervention as a last resort.

The concept of trauma-informed care and recovery from psychiatric illness first emerged in the early 1990s and continues to advance today, buttressed by new findings in developmental neuroscience and recognition of the prevalence of trauma among populations that most frequently access mental health and substance abuse facilities. Much information concerning trauma-informed care continues to be found in the "grey literature" developed by organizations and mental health websites as part of widespread efforts to affect policy on state and local levels (Muskett, 2013).

Trauma may be defined as the personal experience of interpersonal violence, including sexual abuse; physical abuse; severe neglect; loss; and/or the witnessing of violence, terrorism, and disasters (National Association of State Mental Health Program Directors [NASMHPD], 1998). A majority of individuals and children in inpatient behavioral health settings have experienced trauma; consequently, we aim to take universal precautions and presume that every person in treatment has a trauma history. In public mental health settings, as many as 90% of individuals who seek treatment have histories of repeated exposure to trauma and violence; most often beginning in childhood but often continuing to occur in the context of mental health treatment settings (Murphy & Bennington-Davis, 2005).

Issues around seclusion and restraint in behavioral health facilities have been key drivers in the effort to implement trauma-informed care. "To date, the most clearly articulated policy to emerge from the trauma-informed care movement . . . has been the agreement to reduce, and wherever possible, eliminate the use of seclusion and restraint" (Muskett, 2013 p.1). When traumatized patients are restrained or secluded during their hospital stay, they often feel they are being punished, are confused by staff's use of force, do not feel protected from harm, and continue to experience feelings of bitterness and anger for a year or more (NASMHPD, 1998). When a human service program takes the steps necessary to become trauma informed, every part of its organization, management, and service delivery system is assessed and potentially modified to include a basic understanding of how trauma affects the lives of individuals seeking services. In trauma-informed organizations, programs and services are based on understanding the vulnerabilities or triggers of trauma survivors that traditional approaches may exacerbate, so that these services and programs can be more supportive and avoid retraumatization (Jennings, 2007).

Trauma-specific interventions are designed specifically to address the consequences of trauma in the individual and to facilitate healing. Treatment programs generally recognize:

■ the survivor's need to be respected, informed, connected, and hopeful regarding his or her own recovery
■ the interrelation between trauma and symptoms of trauma (e.g., substance abuse, eating disorders, depression, and anxiety)
■ the need to work in a collaborative way with survivors, family and friends, and other human services agencies in a manner that will empower survivors and consumers

Various components in an organization undergo change as it begins to implement recovery and trauma-informed care. Of utmost importance is to seek change from patients on a voluntary, not involuntary, basis. Components of change include listening to staff members; hard-wiring cultural change through policy revision; job descriptions, education, and evaluation; assessing the physical and social environments; adjusting language and vocabulary; and challenging assumptions and expectations (Bennington-Davis, 2010). ZHH has been transforming its model of care to include the principles of recovery and continues to strive to become more trauma informed. "Trauma-informed care is an emerging value that is seen as fundamental to effective and contemporary mental health nursing practice," notes Coral Muskett (2013, p.1). However, as she notes, "Trauma-informed care, like recovery, leaves mental health nurses struggling to transfer these values into day-to-day nursing practice."

Evolution of a Simulation-Based Clinical Skills Course

Although a rich body of literature addresses aggression in behavioral health, there is a dearth of literature on how to educate staff to manage such behaviors. Similarly, despite the wealth of information about psychiatric emergencies and aggression, there is a paucity of literature on the use of simulation in behavioral health. At ZHH, with a view to implementing trauma-informed care, we sought to develop our own clinical skills course to help train UAP. Central to this course was the use of simulation with SPs. In general, SPs portray patients in situations that provide staff members with the opportunity to improve decision-making and problem-solving skills in a safe and nonthreatening environment (Keltner, Grant & McLernon, 2011). Encounters with psychiatric patients, in particular, require subtle empathic skills, and SPs can help staff members practice building alliances with "disturbed and disturbing patients" (Brenner, 2009, p.113). "The presence of real people within scenarios adds to the authenticity of the experience . . . particularly when focusing on patient-centered simulations that emphasize empathy, communication, clinical judgment, and decision making. Using actors is an opportunity for immersive, interactive, and reflective simulation experiences to enhance clinical practice" (Keltner, Grant, & McLernon, 2011, p. 36).

In July 2011 ZHH created a new position, the patient engagement specialist (PES). Under the direction of an RN and the hospital's patient experience program leadership, PESs work with the interdisciplinary treatment teams to engage high-risk patients using crisis prevention/intervention techniques. PESs are unlicensed staff members; the position requires at least 2 years of college in a related field or 6 years of experience in the field of psychiatry as a support staff member, mental health worker, or similar provider. Their backgrounds are varied and multicultural; they range in age from mid-20s to over 60 and offer a wide range of experience. Of the original team, some were mental health workers (behavioral health nursing assistants) who were promoted; three staff members were hired from the outside. Their extensive training during the orientation and probation period focused on verbal de-escalation skills. PES staff members are not assigned to a particular unit; they rotate around the campus to all ten inpatient units. They seek to help patients who are most at risk for aggression or assaultive behavior, proactively interact with them to prevent a crisis or episodes of agitation, and verbally de-escalate during crises. Staff members on the various units, including physicians, nurses, and psychologists, will page PES team members directly when they need assistance in managing an agitated patient; or they may plan in advance to have a PES on the unit if they need to give a patient news that he or she may not want to hear.

As a new post that could put the individuals selected at high risk for violent encounters, we required a specialized training program to provide PES staff members with the skills they needed to perform their job safely. In addition to the standard APT (discussed previously) offered at ZHH, the nursing education and hospital leadership decided to create a simulation program that would allow them to practice and sharpen their skills interacting with extremely agitated patients in an environment that was both safe and as true to the hospital setting as possible. In collaboration with the staff of the NS-LIJ Patient Safety Institute, we developed and piloted the Clinical Skills Course. First offered to PES staff in 2011 we subsequently rolled it out to the rest of the UAP, including mental health workers and psychiatric assistants, in the first quarter of 2012.

With the aid of professional actors as SPs, our mental health workers can train and hone their intervention de-escalation skills, empathizing with and consoling agitated and distressed patients and establishing therapeutic rapport. The objectives of this course are that learners will be able to:

- communicate effectively and therapeutically with mentally ill patients
- decrease episodes of aggression directed toward other patients, staff, and property
- enhance patient and staff safety through improved communication and situational awareness regarding patients' propensity for violence
- understand/empathize with the lived experience of the person experiencing mental illness
- recognize the signs/symptoms of psychiatric distress and intervene most appropriately and efficiently

Sixteen staff members participate in a typical Clinical Skills Course. In groups of four, each member takes part in two back-to-back simulation scenarios with SPs. The scenarios are designed to resemble encounters that a ZHH staff member might experience on a daily basis. A clinical instructor observes each encounter through a one-way glass.

PATIENT #1: "JOANN WARREN"

Female, 35 y.o. Involuntary, new admit from the Emergency Department. Agitated. History of bipolar disorder, currently manic. Spent $50,000 on shopping spree but can't pay her bills. Also has history of cocaine abuse. Husband brought Joann to the ER after she did not pick up kids from school. Refuses to allow search by metal detector or to change into hospital gown.

The staff member enters the room with minimal information—he or she only knows that the patient is newly admitted. "Joann Warren" is manic, agitated, and pacing in the room. The staff member has a single goal: to verbally de-escalate the patient. Joann is very upset that her husband brought her to the hospital; she has flight of ideas and in speech skips from topic to topic. She is sexually provocative toward both male and female staff members and tends to escalate if they allude to her husband or tell her to "calm down" or "relax." (We specifically ask SPs to escalate when a staff member uses these or similar terms, as most patients will do the same.) Staff members attempt to build rapport, allay Joann's concern about her children, and make her feel comfortable with her admission as an inpatient. Each of the several SPs that portrays Joann improvises variations on the bipolar theme. Tactical efforts by staff members to build rapport by talking about her husband backfire because Joann is angry that he brought her to the hospital in the first place. But she usually appreciates it when staff members mention her children; oftentimes that helps begin to build rapport. Similarly, if the staff member tells her directly that she is behaving in an inappropriate manner, she escalates, in the throes of the manic phase of her bipolar disorder, and she does not recognize that her behavior is counterproductive. Every interaction is different in that Joann reacts extemporaneously to what staff members say to her, the words they use, their gestures, and how they act.

PATIENT #2: "WILLIAM CLAY"

Male, 25 y.o., first-break patient, recently returned from Iraq. Diagnosis: schizophrenia and PTSD. He is unpredictable, constantly in others' personal space, with poor boundaries.

Encounters with "William Clay" are generally much more intimidating to staff members. The patient is a war veteran, admitted to the hospital against his will for bizarre and agitated behavior. The staff member in this scenario enters the room to find a patient who is extremely agitated, threatening, cursing and pacing, sometimes banging on cabinets and countertops. William is loud, paranoid, extremely suspicious of anyone with a foreign-sounding name, and difficult to connect with. The staff member's goals are to build rapport and try to calm the patient without telling him how to feel. Staff who put their hands in their pockets or hold them behind their back, or stand too close, tend to escalate William and increase his agitation. Staff members can be successful in this scenario if they manage to get William to sit in a chair and lower his voice. Those best able to build rapport validate his feelings about returning from war. Staff members who have a military history tend to be successful, but those who try to fabricate one often find themselves on a slippery slope. William, a savvy veteran who usually figures out when a staff member is not being truthful, provides an important lesson when staff recognize that they can potentially damage the therapeutic relationship they were trying to create if he loses trust in them.

Post hoc, the SPs assess staff members' de-escalation efforts in several areas from the perspective of the role they played. We created a checklist (Figure 13.1) that they use to evaluate staff performance, and they are also able to add comments. This tool allows us to pinpoint areas in which employees may need to do further work and, if necessary, helps to pinpoint the need for additional education.

Checklist Response
(Group By Students)

INSTITUTE NAME   : North Shore LIJ
NAME   : William Clay
STUDENT ID   :   Date: 6/11/2013-1

CASE: Michael Harris
Comment: *She remained calm & allowed me my own time to calm down by her tonality; she had 2 American flags on her name tag, which let me feel she was on "our side". But I still didn't feel confident enough to allow her to help me. She made no promises (calling Homeland Security. If she said something to reassure me that secutiry measures would be taken ay my "office" I would've felt safe enough to open up more & trust her.*

CATEGORY: SP IPS-Comm   Evaluator: —

Q.	Question Text	Response
1	Did the staff member wash/sanitize their hands before and after shaking your hand?	Poor
2	Did the staff member present his/her self in a professional manner; appropriate dress and grooming?	Good
3	Did the staff member introduce him/her self as a Mental Health Worker?	Fair
4	Did the staff member communicate therapeutically (tone of voice soft, doesn't tell you to "relax" of "calm down"?)	Fair
5	Was the staff member empathetic (stages "i understand," or "i would feel like that too," etc.?)	Fair
6	Did the staff member treat you courteously and with dignity avoiding patronizing attitudes?	Fair
7	Did the staff member establish proper spacing and protective distance with the patient?	Good
8	Did the staff member consistently demonstrate engaging body language through out the interview?	Fair
9	Did the staff member ask open-ended questions regarding present illness?	Poor
10	Did the staff member show concern for the patients comfort? (All contact with patient is measured and reasonably gentle.)	Fair
11	Did the staff memner demonstrate the ability to verbally de-escalate the patient?	Fair

CASE: Joanne Warren
Comment: *she spoke to me respectfully aside from asking me to lower my voice about 3 times. I did feel as if she was listening to me, but she was also trying to let me know the facts of what was going to go on here. I did not like that she continuously brought up my husband, and even laughed at one point when I refetrred to him using a not so nice term. She seemed to really want to help me in regards to getting me help. She was not rude at any point, and her spacing was not threatening.*

CATEGORY: SP IPS-Comm   Evaluator: —

Q.	Question Text	Response
1	Did the staff member wash/sanitize their hands before and after shaking your hand? Comment: *N/A*	Fair

FIGURE 13.1 Arcadia Checklist.
Standardized Patients evaluate staff performance with a checklist and written comments. Reproduced by courtesy of Education Management Solutions, Inc.

In addition, after each simulation encounter, a debrief takes place with the SP, the staff member, and the clinical instructor who observed the scenario. We employ the "debriefing with good judgment" approach developed by Rudolph and colleagues (2006) that encourages instructors to style interventions in terms of advocacy and inquiry (see Chapter 2), with the aim of developing constructive critiques that staff members can appreciate and assimilate. Debriefing needs to be psychologically safe and staff members need to feel free to explore and try new things, and experience trust and support in an adult educational context.

Narrative Pedagogy

During sessions of the clinical skills class, with only four staff members engaged in simulation at one time, the remaining 12 participate in ancillary educational activities. With a focus on patient stories and experiences, these activities aim to help staff members develop and articulate empathy and the skills associated with successful de-escalation without the use of force or coercion. For this element of experiential learning, located squarely in the affective domain, as methodology we employ narrative pedagogy—that is, we examine patients' real stories to understand the challenges that they face in contending with mental illness. As Walsh describes it, "Narrative pedagogy requires teachers and students to work together to arrive at a shared understanding of the meaning of the patient/nursing staff story . . . This approach can lead to stories acting as catalysts for the exploration of topics that are very difficult to discuss . . . and provides an opportunity for patients and their families to have their voices heard and brought into focus as their story is told . . . it facilitates the preparation of students for exposure to the reality of practice and allows them to begin to rehearse strategies for coping with the emotional demands of their work" (Walsh, 2011, p. 217).

Especially in light of course objectives with respect to empathy and the larger effort to advance toward the trauma-informed care and recovery model, we have found narrative pedagogy to be an ideal tool for use in conjunction with psychiatric simulation. We ask staff members to complete several written activities (Table 13.1) that utilize the narrative approach. In group discussion they read aloud what they have written. We remind them that they should avoid judging their peers, and that the overall goal is one of self-discovery in the service of improving patient care.

Preliminary Results

Experiential learning is more meaningful and adult learners remember more of what they have learned when they have hands-on experience. We find that staff members including UAPs, enjoy the simulation environments. Simulation and associated activities build collegiality, enhance mutual support and trust, and increase staff members' sense of security. Results are difficult to quantify because data in the areas of restraint, seclusion, assaults, and patient satisfaction are confounded by many variables and programs designed to improve the same metrics. Nevertheless, feedback from PESs has been to-date overwhelmingly positive.

TABLE 13.1 Activities: Narrative Pedagogy

■ Write about a time when you were involved in a restraint or crisis episode on your unit
■ Read a story written by a patient about his or her experience in restraints and then write about what you thought about the story
■ Complete a worksheet with "startling statements" that a patient may say to you. Write in your response, and then be prepared to role play with a peer
■ Upon return from your simulation scenarios, write about your experience

Among global assessments: "This is the best class we have ever taken"; "This is so much better than all of the videos we had to watch in orientation"; "Everyone should take this class"; "The nurses need to take this class too"; and "This was the most helpful class we have ever taken." More particularly, PES staff felt that the course enabled them to improve their verbal de-escalation skills.[2] One staff member commented after a recent class, "I was able to get feedback from the SP and now I know what I need to work on. It gave me tips that I can use back at the hospital." In sum, the combination of simulation with SPs and narrative pedagogy appears to be an effective teaching mechanism that can help enable staff members to meet objectives in the affective domain, help them acquire insight into behavior, and improve their empathic connection to patients.The Behavioral Health Clinical Skills course is one facet of an overall patient-centered, trauma-informed care solution. Over several years since its inception, we have been able to significantly decrease our restraint and seclusion rate; the numbers of patient-to-patient assaults have also decreased (Figures 13.2 to 13.4). We cannot cite the clinical skills course as the sole reason for these reductions because the hospital has inaugurated various programs and, in addition, the new inpatient pavilion appears to have had a positive effect on patient satisfaction. These and other factors probably impact the aggression metric. Continued monitoring will allow us to develop more substantive data and further reflection on the efficacy of the course in conjunction with current programming.

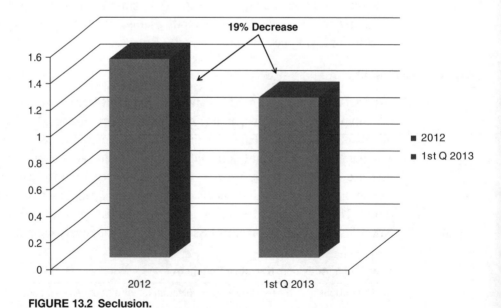

FIGURE 13.2 Seclusion.

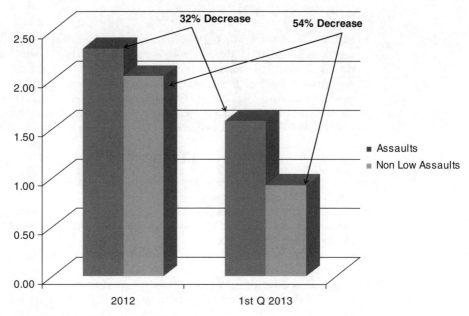

FIGURE 13.3 Patient assaults.

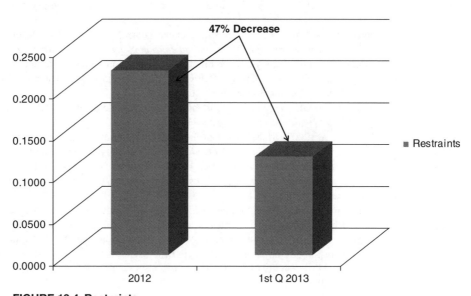

FIGURE 13.4 Restraints.

NOTES

1. PMCS is a comprehensive program developed by New York State to be used in all state psychiatric facilities (2007). The curriculum is made available, free of cost, to other facilities in the state. The APT curriculum content is adapted from PMCS, but is an abbreviated version.
2. As a result of feedback from patient engagement specialists, the course was subsequently provided to the remaining UAPs at ZHH and also offered to mental health workers, psychiatric assistants, and another group of PES staff members at Staten Island University Hospital, Long Island Jewish Hospital and Cohen's Children's Medical Center, all part of NS-LIJ.

REFERENCES

American Psychiatric Nurses Association. (2008). *Position statement on workplace violence.* Retrieved from http://www.apna.org

Bisconer, S. W., Green, M., Mallon-Czajka, J., & Johnson, J. S. (2006). Managing aggression in a psychiatric hospital using a behavior plan: A case study. *Journal of Psychiatric and Mental Health Nursing, 13*, 515–521.

Brenner, A. (2009). Uses and limitations of simulated patients in psychiatric education. *Academic Psychiatry, 33*(2), 112–119.

Champagne, T., & Stromberg, N. (2004). Sensory approaches in inpatient psychiatric settings: Innovative alternatives to seclusion and restraint. *Journal of Psychosocial Nursing, 42*(9),

D'Amico, P., Kim, J., & Stephens, M. (2008). *Aggression Reduction Training.* North Shore Long Island Jewish Health System - The Zucker Hillside Hospital. Unpublished manuscript.

Duxbury, J. (2002). An evaluation of staff and patient views of and strategies employed to manage inpatient aggression and violence on one mental health unit: A pluralistic design. *Journal of Psychiatric and Mental Health Nursing, 9*(3), 325–337.

enotes.com. (2010). *Aggression.* Retrieved from www.enotes.com/gale-psychology-encyclopedia/aggression

Farrell, G., & Cubit., K. (2005). Nurses under threat: A comparison of content of 28 aggression management programs. *International Journal of Mental Health Nursing, 14*(1), 44–53.

Godin, K., Smith, H., Cyr, E., & Finch, K. (2003). Non-violent crisis intervention in Canada. *Mental Health Nursing.* Retrieved from http://www.looksmarthealth.com/p/articles/mi_qa3949/is_200309/ai_n9278361

Irwin, A. (2006). The nurse's role in the management of aggression. *Journal of Pyschiatric and Mental Health Nursing, 13*, 309–318.

Jennings, A. (2007) Models for Developing Trauma-Informed Behavioral Health Systems and Trauma-Specific Services. *An Update of the 2004 Report, Center for Mental Health Services (DMHS), Substance Abuse and Mental Health Services Administration (SAMHSA),U.S. Department of Health and Human Services (HHS).* www.theannainstitute.org/MDT.pdf. Accessed July 2, 2014.

Keltner, N., Grant, J., & McLernon, D. (2011). Use of standardized psychiatric patients: Facilitating success in simulation experiences. *Journal of Psychosocial Nursing, 49*(5), 35–40.

Lepping, P., Steinert, T., Needham, I., Abderhalden, C., Flammer, E., & Schmid, P. (2009). Ward safety perceived by ward managers in Britain, Germany and Switzerland: Identifying factors that improve ability to deal with violence. *Journal of Psychiatric and Mental Health Nursing, 16*, 629–635.

Martin, T., & Daffern, M. (2006). Clinician perceptions of personal safety and confidence to manage inpatient aggression in a forensic psychiatric setting. *Journal of Psychiatric and Mental Health Nursing, 13*, 90–99.

Morrison, EF., & Carney-Love, C. (2003). An evaluation of four programs for the management of aggression in psychiatric settings [Electronic version]. *Archives of Psychiatric Nursing, 17*(4). 146–155.

Murphy, T., & Bennington-Davis, M (2005). *Restraint and seclusion: The model for eliminating their use in healthcare,* Marblehead, MA: HCPro Inc.

Muskett, C. (2013). Trauma-informed care in inpatient menatl health settings: A review of the literature. *International Journal of Mental Health Nursing, 23*(1), 51–59.

National Association of State Mental Health Program Directors (NASMHPD) (1998). Position Statement on Services and Supports to Trauma Survivors. Retrieved http://nasmhpd.org/docs/publications/docs/2008/SRBriefings/I_1_A_NASMHPD_TraumaPositonStatement.pdf

New York State Office of Mental Health. *Preventing and Managing Crisis Situations.* Albany, NY: New York State Office of Mental Health.

Peek-Asa, C., Casteel, C., Veerasathpurush, A., Nocera, M., Goldmacher, S., OHagan, E., & Harrison, R. (2009). Workplace violence prevention programs in psychiatric units and facilities [Electronic version]. *Archives of Psychiatric Nursing, 23*(2). 166–176.

Rudolph, J., Simon, R., Dufresne, R., & Raemer, D. (2006). There's no such thing as "Nonjudgmental" debriefing: A theory and method for debriefing with good judgment. *Simulation in Healthcare: The Journal of the Society for Medical Simulation, 1*(1):49–55.

Spokes, K., Bond., K., Lowe, T., Jones, J., Illingworth, P., Brimblecombe, N., & Wellman, N. (2002). HOVIS—The Hertfordshire/Oxfordshire Violent Incident Study. *Journal of Psychiatric and Mental Health Nursing, 9*, 199–209.

Stubbs, B., Leadbetter, D., Paterson, B., Yorston, G., Knight, C., & Davis, S. (2009). Physical intervention: A review of the literature on its use, staff and patient views, and the impact of training. *Journal of Psychiatric and Mental Health Nursing, 16*, 99–105.

Walsh, M. (2011). Narrative pedagogy and simulation: Future directions for nursing education. *Nursing Education in Practice, 11*, 216–219.

Appendix: Patient Safety, Simulation, and Interprofessional Education Organizations

ORGANIZATION/ ASSOCIATION	DESCRIPTION	FOUNDED	LINK
ECRI Institute	ECRI Institute is an independent, nonprofit organization that studies how to improve the safety, quality, and cost effectiveness of health care. Skilled in applied scientific research, it analyzes medical procedures, devices, drugs, and processes. ECRI disseminates its findings through publishing, education, and consultation.	1968	www.ecri.org
National Patient Safety Foundation (NPSF)	The NPSF is dedicated to improving the safety of patient care. Founded with the support of the American Medical Association, the NPSF is an independent, not-for-profit organization with its own governance structure. It provides an array of resources and support to health care professionals and patients through its online learning, patient safety curricula, research grants, publications, and events, such as promoting Patient Safety Awareness Week.	1997	www.npsf.org
VA National Center for Patient Safety (NCPS)	The NCPS was established to foster a culture of safety throughout the Veterans Health Administration in an effort to prevent and reduce inadvertent harm to patients. The NCPS, one of the pioneers in taking a systems approach to preventing patient injury, has adapted ideas from high-hazard industries to improve health care, including root cause analyses of adverse events; health care failure modes and effect analysis; a national confidential, nonpunitive reporting system; and publication of alerts and warnings. The Center also promotes patient safety research and disseminates information about its programs through an extensive patient-training program, used by VA caregivers as well as professionals from health care organizations across the country.	1999	www.patientsafety.va.gov
The Joint Commission	The Joint Commission accredits health care organizations. An independent, not-for-profit organization, it is widely recognized as the largest, longstanding, national accreditation body. The Joint Commission sets standards for health care quality and encourages organizations to make patient safety a continuous high priority. The Joint Commission establishes and promotes national patient safety goals that influence health care organizations across the country. Its patient safety initiatives include: infection control, sentinel event alerts, and eliminating the use of confusing medical abbreviations.	1951	www.jointcommission.org
Institute for Safe Medication Practice (ISMP)	The ISMP, a 501c(3) nonprofit organization, is dedicated to medication error prevention and safe medication use. It provides a valuable resource to practitioners by gathering data from voluntary reports of medication-related near misses, errors, and adverse events. Based on these reports, ISMP identifies threats to medication safety, alerts practitioners, and disseminates lessons learned to the health care community.	1975	www.ismp.org

Agency for Healthcare Research & Quality (AHRQ)	As part of the U.S. Department of Health and Human Services, the AHRQ sponsors and disseminates research with the goal of improving health care by making it safer, higher quality, more accessible, equitable, and affordable. AHRQ is one of the primary sources for funding patient safety research through its national program of contracts and grants.	1989	www.ahrq.gov
Institute of Medicine (IOM)	The IOM is the health branch of the National Academy of Sciences, one of the National Academies. An independent, nonprofit organization, the IOM prides itself in providing unbiased and authoritative advice to policy makers in government and decision makers in the private sector. Individual IOM members and nonmembers volunteer their knowledge and expertise to conduct studies mandated by Congress or requested by federal agencies and nongovernmental organizations.	1970	www.iom.edu
Institute for Healthcare Improvement (IHI)	The IHI, an independent not-for-profit organization, is dedicated to improving individual and population health. Improving patient safety is one of its five key goals. An innovator in identifying and promoting the implementation of health care improvement, it provides improvement opportunities to frontline health care providers as well as leaders, administrators, and policy makers	1991	www.IHI.org
National Quality Forum (NQF)	The NQF, a nonprofit, nonpartisan, public service organization, focuses on improving the safety, quality, and equity of the health care system by establishing standard measures for evaluating the delivery of health care services. The NQF seeks to establish national priorities for improving health care, collaborating with consumers, clinicians, and purchasers of health insurance.	1999	www.qualityforum.org
National Center for Interprofessional Practice and Education	The National Center for Interprofessional Practice and Education seeks to promote interprofessional education and practice as a viable, efficient, and effective model for delivering health care. The Center aims to foster an integrated redesign of education and clinical practice. It encourages research and serves as a clearinghouse for research findings and for innovative models of practice and education. The Center is based at the University of Minnesota and supported by the Health Resources and Services Administration as well as grants from private foundations.	2012	www.nexusipe.org

ORGANIZATION/ ASSOCIATION	DESCRIPTION	FOUNDED	LINK
Leapfrog Group	The Leapfrog Group brings together organizations that purchase insurance for their employees. Leapfrog seeks to reduce preventable medical error by rewarding hospitals that improve the quality and safety of their patient care. Leapfrog uses the Leapfrog Hospital Survey findings to compare hospitals' performance on national standards and shares the results with consumers and employer insurance purchasers. The Leapfrog Group initiatives are supported by its members as well as the Business Round Table and the Robert Wood Johnson Foundation.	2000	www.leapfroggroup.org
Society for Simulation in Healthcare (SSH)	The SSH is an association of professionals who use simulation for health care education and research. SSH seeks to use simulation to improve patient care by reducing errors and enhancing the performance of clinicians and health care provider teams. SSH members promote the technological development and application of a variety of simulation-based modalities, including manikins (i.e., human patient simulators), virtual reality, standardized patients (i.e., actors representing patients), and task trainers for teaching medical procedures.	2004	www.ssih.org
Anesthesia Patient Safety Foundation (APSF)	The APSF aims to improve the safety of patients undergoing anesthesia. An independent, multidisciplinary organization, the APSF members include clinicians, drug industry representatives, and equipment manufacturers who work together to avoid preventable adverse outcomes for patients. Widely recognized as pioneers in promoting patient safety, the APSF encourages education and research leading to a national exchange of ideas as well as sponsoring patient safety campaigns.	1985	www.apsf.org
American Association of Medical Colleges (AAMC)	The AAMC, a not-for-profit association, represents the academic medicine community, including all the accredited medical schools in the United States and the major teaching hospitals and health systems. As part of its broad mission to support its members' education, research, and patient care activities, the AAMC fosters training in patient safety practices as well as interprofessional education. The AAMC maintains MedEdPORTAL®, a free online source for peer-reviewed educational scholarship, continuing education activities, and innovations to improve patient care. It is developing a similar portal for interprofessional education that will serve as a clearinghouse for learning resources for interprofessional education.	1876	www.aamc.org
Interprofessional Education Collaborative (IPEC)	The IPEC seeks to prepare future health care providers to work collaboratively in team-based patient care. IPEC brings together the associations that represent schools of higher education, in medicine, dentistry, nursing, pharmacy, and public health. IPEC promotes the national exchange of best practices and innovations in interprofessional education. One of its first initiatives was to publish "core competencies" for collaborative, interprofessional practice, designed to guide common curricular innovations among professional schools.	2009	www.ipecollaborative .org

National Committee for Quality Assurance (NCQA)	The NCQA, a private, 501(c)(3) not-for-profit organization, develops and monitors quality standards and performance measures to assess a range of health care settings. The organization's straightforward approach to improving quality is to "Measure. Analyze. Improve. Repeat." Health plans must meet rigorous standards and routinely report on their performance to earn the NCQA's seal of accreditation, indicating that the organization delivers high-quality care and service.	1990	www.ncqa.org
Safe Care Campaign	Inspired by a tragic patient death, this patient-initiated campaign focuses on preventing infections in health care organizations. They have worked with the Centers for Medicare and Medicaid Services to design programs to educate and engage patients in their own care.	2006	www.safecarecampaign.org
Association of Standardized Patient Educators (ASPE)	ASPE is a professional association that fosters the use of standardized patients who are used in medical training to simulate patients in different clinical scenarios. Standardized patients excel in expressing body language, history, physical findings, personality, and emotional characteristics. ASPE advocates the development of this educational methodology by promoting best practices, disseminating research findings, and advancing the skills of its members.	1991	www.aspeducators.org

Index